WHEN SCIENCE
OFFERS SALVATION

WHEN SCIENCE
OFFERS SALVATION

Patient Advocacy and Research Ethics

Rebecca Dresser

OXFORD
UNIVERSITY PRESS
2001

OXFORD
UNIVERSITY PRESS

Oxford   New York
Athens   Auckland   Bangkok   Bogotá   Buenos Aires   Calcutta
Cape Town   Chennai   Dar es Salaam   Delhi   Florence   Hong Kong   Istanbul
Karachi   Kuala Lumpur   Madrid   Melbourne   Mexico City   Mumbai
Nairobi   Paris   São Paulo   Shanghai   Singapore   Taipei   Tokyo   Toronto   Warsaw

and associated companies in
Berlin   Ibadan

Published by Oxford University Press, Inc.
198 Madison Avenue, New York, New York 10016
http://www.oup-usa.org

Library of Congress Cataloging-in-Publication Data
Dresser, Rebecca.
When science offers salvation : patient advocacy and research ethics /
by Rebecca Dresser.
p. cm.   Includes bibliographical references and index.
ISBN 0-19-514313-2
1. Patient advocacy.   2. Medical ethics.   I. Title.
R727.45.D74 2001   174'.2—dc21   00-062388

2 4 6 8 7 5 3 1

Printed in the United States of America
on acid-free paper

To my family

CONTENTS

PREFACE

In 1992, I was invited to participate in a project at the Hastings Center, an institute devoted to the study of bioethics. The project would explore ethical and policy issues raised by the use of long-acting contraceptives. The plan was to follow the standard Hastings Center project model, which included group discussions, individual presentations and papers, and general recommendations for clinical and policy decision making. The model was familiar, for I had been part of several Hastings Center projects investigating other bioethics topics.

The project on long-acting contraceptives had one distinct feature, however. Although the study group would be composed largely of the usual suspects—philosophers, clinicians, public health experts, law professors, social scientists—a few of its members would be community health advocates. Once the meetings started, it became obvious that the group's altered composition would alter the deliberations, as well.

The community health advocates disrupted the ordinary course of business for the project participants. They strayed from the abstract, academic discourse characteristic of the typical Hastings Center inquiry. They disputed scholarly and professional claims by citing real-life situations that exposed gaps in and difficulties with various medical, ethical, and legal approaches. In due course, the other project participants either embraced or discounted the advocacy points of view.

At times, tensions between certain Hastings Center veterans and the newcomers were palpable. Matters came to a head when an elder statesman pronounced the advocates and their supporters confused about their concerns and proceeded to explain what was *really* bothering them! Afterwards, talk arose of dissenting statements and minority reports, topics rarely aired in Hastings Center halls.

Negotiations were painful, and not all were happy with the final product.[1] Yet the process opened my eyes to the advantages of advocacy participation. I found the project meetings more stimulating, wide-ranging, and instructive than any I had experienced. I became convinced that advocates had much to offer the field of bioethics. Here was a group of articulate, knowledgeable, and confident individuals who could bring patients' perspectives to the table. They could offer insights into the personal sides of health problems and the health care system. They could point out weaknesses and omissions in academic and clinical reasoning and, in the process, help keep the bioethics field from becoming stale and complacent.

In the ensuing years, I watched patient advocates become a force in debates over health care policy and practice. Nowhere was their presence more evident than in the realm of biomedical research. When available therapies fell short, as they so often did, advocates found in science the promise of relief— perhaps even full escape—from the burdens of disease. When fate consigned a patient or loved one to serious illness, research advocacy was an uplifting alternative to helplessness and passivity. In their fund-raising and policy work, advocates made research a high priority, in hopes that more science would deliver the solutions they sought. I saw much to admire in the advocates' crusade, but I wondered about the consequences of their high expectations.

This book is my response to the ascent of research advocacy. I have two main objectives. The first is to show how advocacy can enrich and supplement research ethics and policy. Advocates add values and viewpoints missing from scholarly and professional deliberations. They bring fresh interpretations of traditional research ethics principles. Many are also well qualified to participate in research decision making. Although researchers, government officials, and ethicists commonly endorse patient and public participation, not many ordinary people are prepared to enter the world of biomedical science. Because advocates tend to be more informed and assertive than the average citizen, they are more likely to make substantive contributions to research practice and policy.

My second objective is to examine the ethics of research advocacy. Advocates are now major players in the research arena. Their actions affect many people—constituents, other patients, researchers, and the general public. This success brings with it a responsibility to consider the ethical dimensions of their work. Like scientists, physicians, and government officials, research advocates have obligations to probe the full impact of their actions and recommendations. They have obligations to think through how their proposals will affect different groups and individuals over time.

The chapters that follow explore the ethical issues that arise when advocates join in planning, conducting, and evaluating the merits of biomedical research. I investigate ethical questions raised by advocacy campaigns to make experimental interventions more available to seriously ill patients. I describe interest group lobbying for government research funds and consider whether such lobbying enhances or diminishes fairness in funding allocation. I look at two topics relatively low on the advocacy agenda—research ethics oversight and popular reporting about research—and argue that advocates could make substantial contributions in these areas.

The book is intended to serve a variety of readers. Advocates, scientists, and government officials will find material relevant to their work that addresses research design, merit evaluation, priority setting, and ethics oversight. Students and general readers will find information about the biomedical research system, particularly its moral and political dimensions. Patients and other advocacy constituents will find advice on what they should ask of their research advocates, of the scientists and officials traditionally in charge of research, and of the journalists who convey research results to the public. Scholars in bioethics and other academic disciplines will find analysis pertinent to their own writing and teaching projects.

As I worked on this book, biomedical research was constantly in the headlines. Reports of unexpected deaths in gene transfer research elicited from advocates both dismay at the loss of life and pleas to continue the studies.[2] While advocates supported government efforts to publicize opportunities to enroll in clinical trials,[3] federal inspectors expressed ongoing concern about whether the oversight system adequately protects the rights and interests of trial participants.[4] A Massachusetts man who fought to give children with life-threatening conditions access to investigational interventions committed suicide after an experimental measure failed to save his own son.[5]

In these and other events this book describes, we see the complex and competing pressures on contemporary research advocates. We see irresistible hope for research advances and devastating consequences when the advances fail to materialize. We see how advocates' support for research can overshadow their appreciation of the risks and uncertainties inherent in human studies. We see how frustration with the shortcomings of existing medical care drives advocates and many of the rest of us to view research as a more auspicious candidate for financial and emotional investment.[6]

In this book, I focus on the actions and attitudes of advocates, researchers, and government officials. Yet these individuals act with the support of countless others. They express a widely held faith that research will rescue us from the burdens of being human—from the illness, suffering, and death that go along with our status as biological organisms. This book describes some of the human costs of this faith. Reducing these costs will require advocates, scientists, officials, and the rest of us to become more realistic about the sort of salvation that science can offer.

I am grateful to a number of people for their help with this project. Dan Callahan, Nancy King, Carol Levine, Joel Seligman, Carl Wellman, and two anonymous reviewers read all or substantial parts of the manuscript and supplied many good suggestions. Advocate Helen Kornblum was kind enough to take time from her busy schedule to review and comment on several chapters. Thanks also to Dena Davis and Robert Thompson for advice on selected chapters. Karen Black provided thorough and energetic research assistance, and Gary Ellis furnished useful government documents. Cindy Brame and the staff of the Washington University Law Library responded cheerfully and promptly to my numerous requests for assistance. I received financial support for the project from Washington University School of Law.

Discussing segments of the book with a number of groups helped me clarify and refine my ideas. For this, thanks go to faculty and students in the School of Law, School of Medicine, and Department of Philosophy at Washington University in St. Louis. I also benefited from presenting my work at the following conferences: "Bioethics: The Next Twenty-Five Years," University of Tennessee in Knoxville; Faculty of Laws Annual Colloquium, University College, London; American Society of Law, Medicine and Ethics Health Law Teachers Conference; Association for Practical and Professional Ethics Annual Meeting; and the Hastings Center conference on "Biomedical Research: Problems, Possibilities, Puzzles, and Priorities." Last, but definitely not least, thanks to Peter Joy for putting up with me during the months I was preoccupied with this project.

Notes

1. The project yielded two publications. See Ellen H. Moskowitz and Bruce Jennings, eds., *Coerced Contraception? Moral and Policy Challenges of Long-Acting Birth Control* (Washington, DC: Georgetown University Press, 1996); "Long-Acting Contraception: Moral Choices, Policy Dilemmas," *Hastings Center Report* 25 (special supplement, January–February 1995): S1–S32.

2. See statement of Paul Gelsinger and testimony of Eric Kast, Senate Subcommittee on Public Health, Committee on Health, Education, Labor, and Pensions, 2 February 2000, reprinted in *BioLaw* 2 (special supplement, February 2000): S38–S47. See also Deborah Nelson and Rick Weiss, "Patient's Death in Gene Tests Not Reported," *Washington Post*, 3 May 2000, A1.

3. Chapter 3 discusses this development in detail.

4. Department of Health and Human Services Office of Inspector General, *Protection of Human Research Subjects: Status of Recommendations*, OEI-01-97-00197 (Washington, DC: Government Printing Office, 2000).

5. Raphael Lewis and Mac Daniel, "Father of Cancer Victim Kills Himself," *Boston Globe*, 30 April 2000, B1.

6. An example is cancer research advocate Michael Milken's 1999 congressional testimony, in which he criticized the federal government for spending much more on cancer care than it does on cancer research. Senate Subcommittee on Labor, Health and Human Services, and Education, Committee on Appropriations, 16 June 1999. Accessible on the Internet at http://www.senate.gov/~appropriations/labor/testimony/mlkn6_16.htm.

WHEN SCIENCE
OFFERS SALVATION

1

PATIENT ADVOCACY AND THE CHANGING RESEARCH ENVIRONMENT

Today, more than ever, biomedical research is a public affair. Stamps, marches, credit card purchases, designer T-shirts, and Mark McGwire home run balls are vehicles for raising research funds.[1] Celebrities struck by disease start their own foundations to promote the search for a cure.[2] Presidential candidates and congressional leaders pledge to double federal spending for biomedical research.[3] Patient advocacy organizations that once let scientists determine the research agenda now decide for themselves what leads are most promising and award funds to researchers willing to pursue those leads.[4]

The activity goes beyond raising and spending money. A new breed of patient advocate sits at the table with scientists and policymakers, setting research agendas, planning studies, and considering how study results should affect clinical practice. Advocates join scientists evaluating the merit of research proposals that seek government support. Advocates work to expand access to experimental interventions and represent patients and the public in reviewing the ethical dimensions of proposed studies. They supply constituents with information about emerging discoveries and enrolling in clinical trials and have helped fuel a popular media explosion of health research stories.

These developments span many nations. In the United Kingdom, the National Health Service includes advocates in research priority setting and study planning.[5] A French muscular dystrophy organization built its own laboratories and for a time furnished more support for basic human genetics research than did the national government.[6] Wealthy nations sponsoring studies in developing countries recruit community advocates to help plan and conduct the research.[7]

In the United States, advocates' quest for influence over research decision making has changed the politics of biomedical research. Members of Congress and federal agency officials consider advocacy positions when they establish research budgets and policies. Scientific organizations formulating policy positions also consider advocacy perspectives.[8] Researchers share the podium with advocates when they testify at congressional hearings and budget planning sessions. In these settings and elsewhere, advocates challenge researchers to explain and defend their views on which health problems to study and how to study them.

New terms mark the altered power relationships that advocates pursue. Research is planned and conducted by "partnerships," "collaborations," and "coalitions" of scientists, clinicians, and affected communities.[9] People enrolling in studies no longer bear the demeaning label "subject"; instead, they are "participants" or "volunteers" contributing actively and significantly to the research process.[10] Advocates speak not for "timid, passive, horizontal"[11] patients,

5

but for health care "consumers" or "users"[12] who are owed the same high respect and recognition as research professionals conducting important biomedical studies.

Grassroots advocacy is at the heart of many of these developments, and most U.S. grassroots advocates learned their tactics from HIV/AIDS activists. As breast cancer activist Amy Langer told a reporter, "We are absolutely following in the footsteps of the AIDS movement. . . . We've learned that if you want your disease to be dealt with, you go and you talk about it and you market it and you visit and you stomp and you write letters and you do it."[13] In short, passivity and deference to scientific experts and government officials are out; publicity and in-your-face confrontation are in.

Not everyone is thrilled with the changes. Scientists worry that advocates focus too much on cures and treatments without recognizing the importance of basic research as the foundation for clinical applications: "[a]n overly simplistic view of how advances truly occur promises only to stunt the growth of researchers and research areas not capable of immediate great breakthroughs."[14] Researchers also fear that good science will be diluted by extraneous factors, such as the seriously ill patient's desire to "try anything" after conventional therapies have failed: "When the benefits of a new drug or procedure 'make sense' or are 'intuitively obvious,' it becomes difficult or impossible to dampen the enthusiasm of affected patients or interested advocates. . . . [S]erious errors . . . can arise when scientific discipline is not followed."[15]

For their part, public officials are unsettled by the apparent competition among patient advocacy organizations seeking government research dollars:

> There are multiple voices requesting and demanding that more funds be allocated to search for cures for a variety of diseases. Each voice is compelling and each cause deserving. One of the strengths of our system is the freedom of each constituency to make its most compelling case for greater attention and greater resources. But the challenge for our system is to somehow honor and respect those disparate pleas while making the inevitable tough decisions that are required.[16]

Officials and researchers are also concerned that "political correctness" is becoming a dominant force in research priority setting and funding decisions: "It would take a most unscientific credulity to believe that NIH [National Institutes of Health] funding priorities don't reflect a political and media environment."[17]

These pronouncements, to some degree, reflect scientists' and officials' reluctance to share authority in research decision making. Yet the comments also reflect anxiety about ethical and policy issues raised by the new research advocacy. This book examines these ethical and policy issues as they arise in a variety of advocacy contexts.

When advocates help design and conduct studies, they influence what study participants experience and the value of the data that are produced. What role should advocates play in representing the interests of prospective study participants and the interests of the current and future patients who stand to benefit from a study? How much control should advocates exercise in study planning and interpretation?

When advocates work to expand constituents' opportunities to participate in research and to try experimental interventions outside the research setting, they influence what people expect to gain from such interventions. Do advocates' hopes for research advances make them too willing to accept the risks of study participation? Do their positive views of research promote the mistaken belief that participating in a study is equivalent to receiving the best therapy?

When advocates make the case for more research funding for particular health problems, they influence how scarce research resources are distributed. Can lobbying produce a more just allocation of limited research dollars? What gets left out when researchers and officials rely on advocates to provide the "public perspective"?

Embedded in these questions are classic research ethics problems involving the protection of human study participants, the protection of patients from harmful and ineffective treatments, and the just distribution of benefits and burdens produced by biomedical research. Research advocacy presents these questions in novel and subtle ways, however. Many issues remain below the surface, and few have been subjected to explicit analysis.

Research advocacy also brings interest group politics to biomedical research policy. As advocates lobby for funding and policy actions, will biomedical research be increasingly governed by considerations similar to those that govern highway construction and the dairy industry? Will research be diverted from general public health needs and toward the health problems of the wealthy and powerful? If advocacy becomes a major factor in research decision making, can the process be designed to ensure that the interests of disadvantaged groups and individuals are represented?

The new research advocacy is rich with possibility. On one hand, it could contribute to a biomedical research enterprise more in tune with the needs and preferences of the people the enterprise is designed to assist. It could prevent researchers' personal and professional aims from exerting too much control over the research agenda. It could make the potential harms and benefits of research participation less mysterious to and more fairly balanced for people enrolling in studies. It offers fresh opportunities for communication and exchange between scientists and the society they serve, which could give researchers valuable insights into the human side of the problems they study and simultaneously give members of the public a more realistic picture of how research works and what it can achieve.

On the other hand, positive outcomes cannot be guaranteed. Genuine communication between scientists and the public is all too rare. Bridging the gap between the two worlds requires mutual willingness to learn and to value the other's knowledge. If these conditions are unmet, the attempt at dialogue is likely to remain mere window dressing. Shared decision making also costs money, which usually must come from research budgets and the often quite limited funds of advocacy organizations. Some will challenge the use of scarce resources to increase public involvement, and others will try to do it cheaply, thereby elevating the odds against meaningful exchange. Last, we do not know how well government officials, researchers, and advocates will adjust to the altered research environment. Officials will face heightened demands to explain and justify their policy and budget choices. Researchers will be pressed to share power with participant communities and to expand their concept of "good science." Advocates gaining a role in research decision making will become accountable to a public whose needs are more diverse than the advocates' customary constituents. Officials, researchers, and advocates unable to cope with these new responsibilities will decrease the odds of improving research practice and policy.

Recurring Themes

As the opening paragraphs indicated, research advocacy is multifaceted. Advocacy occurs in many different contexts—from the individual research study to the federal budget process. In some settings, advocates are present as a result of vocal public campaigns for inclusion; in others, their involvement is due to regulatory or other policy requirements for public representation. Although research advocacy occurs in multiple settings and circumstances, certain ethical and policy issues are relevant to most advocacy activities. In the chapters that follow, I evaluate advocacy activities in light of five general themes.

First, advocates tend to stress the positive dimensions of the biomedical research enterprise. In much advocacy work, the boundary between research and therapy is fuzzy. The failure to draw a clear line between research and clinical care affects the message advocates communicate to constituents and the broader public.

Many of today's advocates are more interested in expanding opportunities for research participation than in warning constituents of the risks and uncertainties accompanying such participation. Consistent with this approach, advocates often portray study participation as a means to obtain cutting-edge therapy. This characterization of research can promote what is known as the "therapeutic misconception."[18] The therapeutic misconception arises when people confuse the knowledge-seeking mission of research with the patient-centered mission of medicine.

In the medical setting, clinicians practice with the patient's best interests as their principal concern. Treatment recommendations are individualized to reflect the physiologic and other characteristics of a particular patient. In contrast, biomedical research is conducted to produce knowledge for the sake of future patients. Study protocols are designed to collect valid and reliable data, not to furnish the best care to participants. Researchers may *hope* that an investigational agent or procedure will be best for study participants, but in the research phase, the objective basis for this hope is relatively weak.[19] Both safety and effectiveness are less certain than in the medical care arena, where interventions are performed after research has shown them to be reasonably safe and effective. When research and treatment are confused, people may enroll in studies believing that their best interests will guide the investigators' actions. They may harbor unrealistic hope of personal benefit and dismiss the risks and uncertainties accompanying study participation.

Another dimension of the advocacy message is that research can deliver an end to the suffering and deprivation inflicted by illness. Accordingly, much advocacy literature suggests that with more funding for more research we will proceed inexorably "from cause to cure,"[20] eventually winning "the race for the cure."[21] This message may buoy the spirits of people coping with disease and injury and encourage funding as well. The problem is that it also bolsters what law professor Alexander Capron calls the "collective therapeutic misconception."[22] There is no question that research *can* lead to health care improvements. Almost always, however, many years and many false starts occur before practical applications become available. This part of the process is often downplayed in advocacy work; instead, support for research is equated with support for imminent treatment improvements. Research funding is depicted as a way to help people currently burdened by poor health, while an appreciable number of those same people have trouble obtaining the basic, established treatments and services that could extend and improve their lives.

Patient advocates are certainly not to blame for the therapeutic misconception. It is a pervasive notion, long encouraged and condoned by scientists, clinicians, and the popular media. But advocates share some of the responsibility. Moreover, advocates occupy a special position of trust and influence. Representing the interests of constituents may require of them a less enthusiastic, more cautionary approach than is common.

Advocates' perspectives on research quality is a second theme relevant to the new research environment. In measuring research quality, advocates tend to focus on a project's ability to benefit people affected by or at risk for health problems. When they contribute to research planning and priority setting, advocates emphasize the real-life effects of biomedical science. For example, advocates on an advisory committee to the Department of Defense Program for Breast Cancer Research helped establish a custom of starting meetings "with a moment of silence dedicated to a person who is living with or who has died from breast cancer."[23]

Although biomedical research has always had improved health as its over-arching aim, research advocacy highlights and reinforces this aim. The emphasis on concrete benefits can enhance or diminish the value of research. On the positive side, advocates can keep scientists from becoming too detached from the ultimate goal of biomedical research. They can prevent investigators from becoming so caught up in the elegance of science that they lose sight of what patients actually need and how those needs might be met. They can discourage government officials from funding research that primarily satisfies scientific curiosity and advances professional goals.

At the same time, advocates can be so focused on producing health benefits that they end up impeding this process. Advocates can encourage Congress to set aside large portions of research budgets for narrowly targeted studies, leaving too little for the basic science that underlies much clinical progress. They can promote policies and practices that expand constituents' access to unproven interventions at the cost of prolonging or preventing the research necessary to determine whether those interventions are safe and effective.

Biomedical science is being "democratized" through the work of research advocates. As philosopher of science Nancy Maull observes, advocacy can "get us thinking about how science might be different and under what circumstances difference would mean improvement."[24] Advocacy emerges out of and underscores the human-centered essence of biomedical science. It raises basic questions about the importance of different kinds of knowledge and about who is qualified to decide what knowledge is important. It raises questions about the nature of research expertise and the weight that potential health impact should carry in research merit evaluations. Determining when different science means better science requires decision makers to distinguish genuine desires to safeguard research quality from the habits and other less worthy motivations that can underlie opposition to change.

The uneven quality and legitimacy of representation is the third theme relevant to research advocacy. Many research advocates are activists speaking for people with a particular disease or injury. Activists frequently assume this role on their own initiative. They volunteer for a patient advocacy organization and eventually enter the research arena as a lobbyist, spokesperson, or study adviser. Many advocates have a close personal connection to the group they represent in that they are themselves affected by the relevant condition or have a close relative who is affected.[25]

Not all research advocates fit this mold, however. Another kind of advocate is the community leader called on to represent a specific population whose members will be asked to participate in research—usually people in a particular geographic location or people identifying with a particular ethnic group. A third category of advocate is the clinician who cares for patients with the condition of interest or who lives and works in the community where research will be performed. A fourth variation is the researcher who studies a condition and joins in lobbying for research funding or policy actions relevant to people with the disease. Individuals occupying these different categories bring different loyalties and world views to their advocacy work. Officials and researchers can influence the content of advocacy by choosing representatives from one of these categories.

Advocacy contributions are affected by the contact a representative has with constituents, as well. Some advocates receive direct guidance from constituents. Others appear to take positions based primarily on assumptions about constituent interests. Some advocates are "lay experts"[26] who are extremely well-informed about the scientific, medical, and social dimensions of the relevant health problem. Others rely on knowledge acquired through personal experiences with illness. Advocates are not always accountable to a particular constituency, and some appear to operate free of organization-imposed constraints. It also appears that few advocates are chosen by election or other democratic processes. Individual advocates thus vary in their abilities and qualifications to act as a particular group's representative in research decision making.[27]

The problem of group or community definition also pervades research representation. Sometimes it is difficult to determine who should be included as members of the population that will be affected by a research decision. Sometimes the population is quite diverse and includes people with very different economic, social, and personal concerns. Sometimes patients' families have interests that deviate from, and even conflict with, patients' interests. Sometimes organizations claiming to represent the same population take opposing positions on research issues. Sometimes no organization exists to advocate on behalf of affected individuals, or the one that exists lacks the staff or resources required to participate. When these difficulties are present, research representation can become complex and contested.

The fourth theme is fairness in research advocacy. Advocacy is designed to ensure that the values and preferences of people affected by or at risk for health problems are at the forefront when research decisions are made. But again, the diversity of this group—which in its broadest sense includes everyone—means that its members may have widely varying values and preferences. And in many research contexts, individual patients and groups of patients have competing or conflicting interests. Individuals and groups lacking an advocate at the table may lose out when important research choices are made. Unless care is exercised, measures aimed at increasing fairness in research decision making can instead produce substantial unfairness.

Achieving fairness in research advocacy requires attention to process. When officials and researchers consider only the views of advocates initiating contact and exerting pressure, studies and policies fail to take into account the interests of patients whose advocacy organizations lack the necessary expertise or resources to be proactive. In these circumstances, studies and policies also fail to take into account the interests of people unrepresented by any advocacy organization. When officials and researchers simply create opportunities for advocates to communicate their views or join research planning and policy projects, patients represented by organizations with the most resources are the primary beneficiaries. Thus, to promote genuine fairness in research decision making, affirmative outreach and financial support must accompany opportunities for research advocacy.

The sheer number of affected groups with a stake in research decisions also creates fairness issues. In many research contexts, practical limits exist on the number of constituencies that can be directly represented. For example, when the director of the NIH, the major government funding agency for biomedical research, assembles a council of public representatives to "bring public views to NIH activities, programs, and decision-making,"[28] only a few of the numerous interest groups can have a representative appointed. These practical constraints create a need for fair procedures governing representative selection and for supplementary mechanisms to elicit the views of affected groups not directly represented in a particular research activity.

Fairness also depends on officials' and researchers' responses to patient advocates. Fairness is not promoted when officials and researchers smile and listen, then ignore, patient advocates. Fairness is enhanced when the decision-making process includes features to ensure that advocates' views are taken seriously. Such features include requirements to prepare written explanations for research policy decisions and, in some situations, to offer advocates an opportunity to argue in favor of revisions.

A fifth theme is the connection between research advocacy and research ethics. In the United States, the Belmont Report[29] stands as the most eloquent and enduring articulation of research ethics principles. The report was issued in 1979 by the National Commission for the Protection of Human Subjects of Biomedical and Behavioral Research. Congress established the commission in the wake of publicity about unethical research practices, most notably by Public Health Service researchers studying syphilis in rural Alabama. In this study, investigators withheld effective treatment from nearly four hundred African American men without their knowledge or consent.[30]

The Belmont Report sets forth three ethical principles to guide human studies. One principle addresses respect for persons. According to Belmont, we show respect for persons by honoring their informed and voluntary choices. If internal impairments or external conditions compromise their ability to exercise free and informed choice, we respect them by protecting them from harm.

In research, the investigator shows respect for persons by giving prospective participants the facts they need to make an informed choice about study enrollment and by refraining from using coercion or highly tempting incentives to elicit their consent. To show respect for individuals lacking decisional capacity (such as children or people with dementia), the investigator studies such individuals only after a parent, close relative, or other appropriate surrogate makes an informed and voluntary decision to permit enrollment. Investigators also show respect by proceeding only as long as the decisionally incapable individual assents (expresses a willingness to participate) and study discomforts and risks are limited.

Another Belmont principle addresses beneficence. This principle calls for researchers to maximize potential benefits and minimize risks accompanying both specific studies and the broader research enterprise. Investigators must reduce study risks to the minimum level consistent with obtaining the desired scientific information. Any remaining risks must be outweighed by potential benefits to participants, if any, and by the contribution that study findings could make to future health care improvements.

Belmont's final principle emphasizes justice in distributing research burdens and benefits. Investigators ought not rely disproportionately on certain individuals and groups to be research participants. This form of injustice was common before the 1970s, when researchers often conducted studies on poor, uneducated, and otherwise vulnerable people.[31] The justice principle also holds that individuals and groups should receive a "fair share" of the treatment and other benefits flowing from research. This principle may be violated when studies fail to include women, children, older people, or other populations whose biological characteristics or social circumstances might affect study findings. For members of these groups to enjoy the benefits produced through research, some must be included as study participants. Thus, the justice principle counsels against unfairly including *or* excluding people as study participants.

The Belmont Report principles underlie the regulatory policy that governs federally, and a substantial portion of privately, funded research in the United States.[32] The principles guide the decisions of ethics review committees (known in the United States as institutional review boards) evaluating proposals for human studies. International research ethics statements, including the Nuremberg Code and the Helsinki Declaration, endorse principles similar to those in the Belmont Report. Many nations also have incorporated such principles into their domestic policies.[33]

Though widely supported and highly influential, the Belmont Report principles leave many contemporary research ethics problems unresolved. Biomedical research has grown and changed since the Belmont Report and the U.S. oversight system came into being. More research is conducted, and industry sponsors an increased portion of it.[34] Research ethics questions arise in a wider variety of public policy areas. Research in certain areas, such as genetics, presents novel questions about who is vulnerable to research harms and whose permission is required to conduct a study. Current pressures to increase access to investigational interventions raise questions not fully addressed by the Belmont Report and the existing regulations on protection of research participants.

The research ethics field has grown and changed as well. Today's scholars and clinicians are dissatisfied with existing research ethics tools. A sense has arisen "that the conceptual and regulatory framework for attention to ethics in research with human subjects is insufficiently rich and nuanced to be helpful in addressing certain key pervasive ethical issues."[35] Ethicists thus seek inspiration from feminist[36] and narrative[37] ethics, from empirical study of actual research experiences,[38] and from the life stories of people whose illnesses led them into the world of clinical research.[39]

Research advocacy presents scholars and clinicians with another opportunity to extend ethics analysis. Many advocates are exquisitely familiar with the desires, fears, and vulnerabilities experienced by both people considering study participation and patients who stand to benefit from research advances. Many advocates know what it is like to decide whether to enter a randomized clinical trial that will expose them to uncertain risks and benefits. Many are well situated to determine the information people need to make such choices and effective ways of delivering that information. Advocates also have knowledge that bears on whether a study's potential benefits outweigh its risks. They possess insights into whether a policy or practice may produce an unfair distribution of research burdens and benefits, as well. In short, many advocates are committed, energetic, thoughtful, and articulate individuals possessing knowledge relevant to research ethics and policy questions. They can help fill gaps left by the existing ethical and regulatory framework, point to unrecognized problems with accepted ethics positions, and supply personal knowledge often missing from standard ethics analysis.

Advocacy organizations also can be a vibrant political force against research abuses. As early as 1949, Dr. Leo Alexander made this observation in his classic article about the Nazi era, "Medical Science Under Dictatorship."[40] Alexander described as a promising development "the societies of patients afflicted by various chronic diseases that have recently sprung up." He believed these groups could effectively counteract medical and societal tendencies to devalue the lives of such patients. He saw patient organizations as "having an extremely wholesome effect in introducing fresh motivating power into the ivory towers of academic medicine," as well as "an assertion of democratic vitality" reminding physicians of their moral responsibilities to protect people affected by disease and disability from unethical research and harmful social policies. In the years since Alexander's article, however, ethicists have for the most part failed to recognize this important advocacy role and have given inadequate thought to how advocacy groups might help resolve ethical and policy problems in contemporary biomedical research.

Related to these issues is the relationship between patient advocates and professional ethicists. Scholars and clinicians making a living in the bioethics field often see themselves, and are seen by others, as patient and public representatives in research decision making. Now patient advocates are increasingly assuming this role. Where do the two groups find common cause and where do they part ways? What considerations should guide ethicist–advocate relationships?

Advocacy in Context

The remainder of this book examines patient advocacy in various research settings. Chapter 2, Advocates on the Research Team—Shaping and Assessing Science, considers advocacy primarily in the context of individual research studies. The U.S. pioneers in this form of advocacy were HIV/AIDS and breast cancer activists. At the international level, the participatory research movement began in the 1970s to urge active involvement of local community members in planning and conducting studies.

Advocates representing many disease constituencies are now engaged in planning, conducting, and evaluating the results of research. They also serve on committees that assess the merit of proposed studies seeking government support. Involving advocates in these activities can have positive outcomes in the form of more meaningful, more ethical, and more efficient research. On the other hand, their involvement has the potential to disrupt long-standing scientific and academic traditions, compromise advocates' ability to represent their constituents, and, in the worst-case scenario, sanction unethical research practices.

The next four chapters address advocacy in broader policy contexts. Chapter 3, Hope Versus Hypothesis Testing: Expanded Access to Experimental Interventions, considers advocacy efforts to expand constituents' opportunities to try investigational drugs and other novel interventions. HIV/AIDS advocates were instrumental in convincing federal officials to adopt rules making unapproved agents more widely available to seriously ill people. Some, though not all, women's health advocates promoted widespread access to bone marrow transplants for women with advanced breast cancer before the procedure's safety and effectiveness had been demonstrated. Advocates representing a variety of constituencies conducted successful campaigns to alter policies and practices that kept women and people in certain age and ethnic groups from participating in research.

Advocates at times have good reason to promote expanded access to experimental interventions. In certain circumstances, however, expanded access comes at the cost of research participants' and patients' welfare. Advocates who place undue emphasis on access can promote confusion between insufficiently studied interventions and accepted health care, with negative consequences at both the individual and societal levels. A fixation on access can also substantially increase the costs to society of determining whether a new agent or procedure carries unjustifiably high risk or is relatively ineffective.

In the next two chapters, I turn to the problem of allocating limited resources for biomedical research. Chapter 4, Fairness in Allocating Government Research Funds, examines how Congress and the NIH distribute federal funds for biomedical research. Officials at NIH consider several substantive criteria, such as public health needs and scientific opportunity, in deciding how to apportion research funds. Certain members of Congress and patient advocates have criticized agency officials, however, for failing to apply these criteria in a systematic manner. These critics argue that, in reality, scientists and the most politically savvy advocacy organizations exert substantial control over how public research funds are divided. Critics want the NIH to adopt a more transparent allocation process that allows others to evaluate how well the formal priority-setting criteria are being met. Distributive and procedural justice principles support certain revisions in the agency's approach to funding allocation.

Chapter 5 explores one such revision in detail. Public Participation in Allocating Government Research Funds describes recent NIH efforts to expand opportunities for patient advocates to be involved in research priority setting. The changes were a response to findings that the agency had not done enough to solicit information from individuals and organizations with interests in how research funds are allocated.

Giving patient advocates a greater role in biomedical research priority setting could make federal spending more responsive to public preferences and interests. But giving advocates more influence could also heighten funding inequalities, further politicize funding decisions, and promote federal budgets that shortchange other areas of science as well as health care, housing, and other social programs. Applying principles of deliberative democracy to research priority setting can help avoid these outcomes.

In chapter 6 I turn to policies calling for members of the general public to participate in decision making about research ethics. Advocates in Research Ethics Oversight: A Voice for the Public? considers the increasingly common practice of involving the public in ethics review. In the United States, this practice began with the Federal Policy for the Protection of Human Subjects, which required appointment of public members to institutional review boards evaluating the ethics of proposed human studies.[41] It continued with federal provisions exempting studies of potential emergency interventions from ordinary consent requirements. Investigators seeking exemptions must meet conditions intended to substitute for the usual consent rules. One such condition is to inform and consult with people from "the communities in which the clinical investigations will be conducted and from which the subjects will be drawn."[42]

Community participation is a part of research ethics oversight in other nations as well. When developed nations sponsor research in developing countries, investigators are advised to submit their studies for ethics review by people "thoroughly familiar with the customs and traditions of the [local] community."[43] Leaders of ethnic and religious groups also recommend that investigators and review committees consult with group representatives about the ethics of study proposals. These leaders propose community consultation for studies that expose particular ethnic or indigenous groups to discrimination or stigma (for example, a study on a possible genetic predisposition to alcohol abuse).[44]

Such policies and proposals raise a number of questions. What are the justifications for requiring public participation in ethics oversight? Do public members on research ethics review committees provide effective representation? What characteristics of the review system diminish the public participant's ability to contribute? Greater participation by patient advocates could strengthen the public voice in research ethics oversight.

When advocates enter the research policy arena, they bring opinions shaped by popular media accounts of biomedical research. Chapter 7, Advocacy for Accuracy in Research Reporting, considers the "breakthrough mentality" that characterizes much popular media coverage. Reporters and the scientists they interview are prone to exaggerate the clinical implications of research findings. But those indulging in overstatement violate professional responsibilities to tell the truth to patients and the public. By speaking out against sensationalism, advocates can discourage misleading reports about research results. By taking advantage of the burgeoning information available on the Internet and elsewhere, advocates can direct constituents and the public to accurate and realistic research accounts.

Chapter 8, Research Advocacy Today and Tomorrow, reexamines the five broad themes raised by research advocacy. I propose ethical principles for research advocacy, urge greater collaboration between advocates and ethicists, and describe three challenges facing future advocates: 1) determining whether HIV/AIDS activism should continue to serve as the model for research advocacy, 2) responding to the rise of industry-sponsored clinical research, and 3) formulating positions on xenotransplantation, stem cell research, and other novel research interventions.

Language and Point of View

Readers will find in this book a variety of terms that refer to individuals involved in research advocacy. I use the terms *patient advocate*, *research advocate*, and *activist* to describe an individual—usually a layperson—acting on behalf of constituents affected by specific health problems. I use the term *representative* to refer either to an advocate serving a specific disease or demographic constituency or to someone designated to speak for the general public. Other terms for people in these positions crop up, such as *consumer*, *lay representative*, and *community consultant*. Because I dislike the passivity associated with the term *research subject*, I use *research participant* to refer to people from whom research data are collected. I depart from this practice when referring to sources incorporating the traditional term *research subject*.

My approach to this analysis is from the vantage point of someone trained in law and bioethics. I have spent most of my working life teaching medical and law students about bioethics, including research ethics and policy. As an ethicist, I bring awareness of the strengths and weaknesses of the conventional research ethics framework, and as a lawyer, I bring a focus on fair procedures and familiarity with the regulatory system.

I have served on institutional review boards, NIH research merit review panels, and an NIH institute advisory council. These experiences awakened my interest in research advocacy. They also shaped my ideas about what advocacy can contribute to research decisions and where advocacy can fall short. As someone with little scientific training, I appreciate both how difficult and how rewarding it can be to bring the "outside" perspective to research decision making. I have talked often with others—advocates, clinicians, ethicists, scientists, and government officials—about what it might mean to represent the public in various research settings.

Finally, I offer this analysis in the spirit of discovery. Research advocacy creates a wealth of new issues and great potential for change. My overall goals are to describe the emergence of advocacy in various settings, to delineate the questions and problems it raises, and to offer ideas on how to proceed. I also attempt to point out areas in which advocates and researchers share common goals, where they part ways, and how they might achieve maximal accommodation of each other's views.[45] In doing so, I hope to help advocates, researchers, and officials with the work they are doing. I hope that this material will stimulate them to think systematically and creatively about what they can do to promote ethical and effective advocate involvement in research decision making.

I hope as well to give scholars a closer look at the advocacy phenomenon and to build a foundation for future inquiry. Research advocacy is a phenomenon ripe for interdisciplinary analysis by scholars of political science, philosophy, history, anthropology, and sociology, to name a few. I consider this book a first take and look forward to what others have to say about this fascinating feature of the contemporary research landscape.

2
ADVOCATES
ON THE
RESEARCH TEAM—
SHAPING AND
ASSESSING SCIENCE

In the first decade of the disease the medical establishment produced only one treatment drug, AZT, at a cost of over one billion dollars. . . . The solution to this deficiency was obvious: the community's own empowerment by way of decisionmaking in *all* aspects of clinical trials and medical research.[1]

Not only do consumer participants return to their communities and report about the peer review process thus fostering understanding and communication between scientists and the general public, their presence during the review serves to remind basic scientists of the human component of this disease and the need for more research on psychological and social aspects, and health care delivery.[2]

[R]esearch is all too often done on participants, rather than with or by them.[3]

Advocates want a say in the way biomedical research is conducted. In the United States, HIV/AIDS and breast cancer advocates were the first to make this demand. In Britain, Canada, and some developing countries, it arose with the participatory research movement, which promotes community involvement in health research. By the late 1990s, advocates representing a multitude of patient and community groups wanted research to reflect their judgments on which conditions should be studied and which study methods adopted. They wanted a role in interpreting, publicizing, and applying study results. And they wanted to help decide which research proposals merited government funding.

Ethical and scientific aims can be advanced by integrating advocacy views into decisions about study design, procedures, and merit. Achieving genuine integration is no simple matter, however. Attempts to make advocates part of the research team often collide with scientific tradition and the research establishment. Moreover, although the approach offers benefits to patients and society, when advocates join the research team, new risks and complications arise both for advocates and for their constituents.

Origins

A look at advocacy activities in three contexts illustrates how advocates can change research practices. In the United States, HIV/AIDS activists were leaders in challenging the research status quo. During the 1980s, as gay men sought to cope with a growing epidemic, they looked to medicine for assistance. Because physicians and scientists could tell them little about the new disease, the need for research was obvious. Activists initially campaigned for more resources and a heightened national commitment to study the condition. Once funding was secured and research under way, however, advocates rebelled against much of what they saw.

The focus of activist discontent was the randomized clinical trial (RCT). The RCT is commonly regarded as the gold standard for determining whether an experimental drug or other intervention is good enough to enter the realm of accepted therapy. Participants in an RCT are randomly assigned to different study groups. To keep participants' and researchers' expectations from influencing experimental results, study group assignments are usually concealed until data collection is complete. Typically, one group receives a new (but still experimental) agent, while the other receives an available standard treatment.

The experimental agent's effects are then compared with those of the standard treatment to determine which agent is more effective and produces the least serious side effects or other complications.[4]

Often, one group in an RCT is assigned to receive a placebo, an agent believed to have no direct effect on the condition being studied. Sometimes, health improvements occur simply because study participants believe they are receiving something more effective for their disease—the so-called placebo effect. Adding a placebo group allows scientists to separate the improvements produced by the experimental and other active agents under study from any improvements caused by the placebo effect.[5]

To the HIV/AIDS activists, many of the RCT conventions seemed shockingly inhumane. In their eyes, it was unethical to give anyone with a life-threatening disease an inactive agent or a relatively ineffective standard treatment instead of a promising new experimental agent. They attacked other dimensions of the RCT as well. People with HIV/AIDS often were told that during clinical trial participation they would have to refrain from taking other medications, including drugs designed to relieve symptoms unrelated to the study. Others were excluded from trials because their past medication use might improperly influence study findings.[6] Scientists claimed that excluding these individuals would make it easier to isolate the effects of the test drugs.

Activists discovered that they had to become familiar with scientific concepts to argue effectively against the RCT's rigid rules. Lay advocates proceeded to learn "the language of the journal article and the conference hall."[7] They became sufficiently knowledgeable to question what they saw as unnecessarily restrictive research methods and to invoke the arguments of mainstream scientists dubious about the need for such methods. Lay advocates were joined by clinicians from the gay community, who added credibility to the challenge.

Activists eventually were able to buttress their ethical criticisms with scientific and practical arguments against the standard RCT approach. They persuaded researchers that some restrictive RCT demands could be loosened without undermining the scientific value of the findings. For example, they convinced scientists to expand eligibility criteria by arguing that study results would be more applicable to the general population of people with HIV/AIDS if a more diverse and hence more representative group participated.[8]

Practical impediments to conducting HIV/AIDS research also lent authority to the activists' claims. Many HIV-positive people refused to participate in studies if there was a chance they would receive a placebo or a standard therapy they deemed unsatisfactory. Many also were unwilling to stop taking other drugs while they participated in research. Some people entering studies later became "noncompliant"—a term activists rejected because it implied that participants should be subservient to the wishes of the scientists conducting a trial. "Noncompliant" participants gave inaccurate reports of past medication use, continued to take other drugs during a trial, dropped out of studies if they perceived no improvement in their conditions, and shared what they guessed was the promising experimental agent with other study participants who believed they were receiving only placebos. Thus, activists could make a compelling case that trials would be impossible to conduct unless RCT rules were modified.

Ultimately, advocates for people with HIV/AIDS changed conventional clinical trial practices and, in the process, taught scientists to see them as essential research contributors. Sociologist Steven Epstein summed up the activists' achievements as follows:

> The arguments of AIDS activists have been published in scientific journals and presented at scientific conferences. . . . Their arguments have brought about shifts of power between competing visions of how clinical trials should be conducted. Their close scrutiny has encouraged basic scientists to move compounds more rapidly into clinical trials. And their networking has brought different communities of scientists into cooperative relationships with one another. . . . [9]

Breast cancer activists, too, had a major impact on U.S. research. Quick to learn from their counterparts in the HIV/AIDS community, breast cancer activists began in the early 1990s to demand a greater role in the research process. At first, their influence was most visible in the Department of Defense (DOD) Program for Breast Cancer Research. In 1993, advocates convinced Congress to set aside $210 million of the DOD budget for breast cancer research. Because DOD was not a traditional biomedical research sponsor, the agency lacked established conventions for determining which studies it would fund. Activists saw this as an opportunity for a fresh approach, one that included advocates from the very beginning.[10] The system that emerged gave advocates a role in determining the overall goals of the DOD program as well as the proposals that received funding.

In the DOD program, research proposals requesting funding are reviewed at two levels. Merit review panels conduct the initial evaluation. Each panel has 15–20 members, including 2 consumers, defined as individuals diagnosed with breast cancer and nominated by breast cancer organizations. Consumers who seek to serve must submit applications, which include essays describing their ability to contribute to the review process. Although consumers and scientists are assigned slightly different roles in proposal review, the votes of consumers and scientists count equally in assigning merit scores to proposals.[11] Consumers with scientific training are appointed to panels that consider proposals outside their fields, "to avoid confusion between the 'science' and 'advocacy' roles."[12]

At least three or four consumers serve on a separate integration panel, which sets broad research goals for the program. This group also acts as a second-level review panel for research proposals. Here, final recommendations for funding are made based on the proposals' merit scores and their potential contributions to the program's overall goals.[13] At this level, the definition of consumer expands to include people in families at high risk for breast cancer and "others with specific interests and perspectives related to breast cancer."[14] Scientists qualifying as consumers "are asked to function as either a scientist or a consumer, but not both."[15]

In 1997, the DOD program was evaluated by a committee of the Institute of Medicine, a federal advisory organization. According to the committee, "most observers have found the participation of consumers to be a very positive aspect of the . . . peer review process, and one that may serve as a model for other peer review systems."[16] This positive evaluation of consumer participation was confirmed in 1999, when a patient advocate was elected chair of the integration panel.[17]

Breast cancer activists promoted consumer involvement in other research programs as well. In 1994, in response to advocacy efforts, the Department of Health and Human Services brought together public agencies and private organizations to formulate a National Action Plan on Breast Cancer. One goal of the plan is to "ensure culturally appropriate consumer involvement at all levels in the development, implementation, and communication of . . . research studies. . . ."[18]

Activists also created a training program to give patient advocates the sort of scientific knowledge that enabled HIV/AIDS activists to gain the respect of biomedical researchers. Each year, the National Breast Cancer Coalition's Project Leadership Education and Advocacy Development (LEAD) sponsors intensive courses covering cancer biology, genetics, epidemiology, and the research funding process. Refresher courses are available at a yearly advocacy training conference, and advocates can keep up with scientific developments by participating in the organization's journal club.[19]

At the international level, the coalition organized a series of conferences to promote and strengthen advocacy efforts worldwide. In 1999, conference participants adopted as a global priority "[i]ncreasing government-funded research into the causes of and cure for breast cancer, with breast cancer advocates integrally involved in that process."[20]

A separate international development is the participatory research movement, which supports community involvement in planning, conducting, and acting on health research. More overtly political than the HIV/AIDS and breast cancer advocacy movements, participatory research has roots in critical social, feminist, and phenomenological theories about oppression and empowerment.[21] In essence, the approach exhorts researchers to relinquish their usual control over the study process and to share power with prospective study participants.

Participatory research holds that members of the study population possess knowledge that is as essential to a project's success as is the scientific and medical knowledge researchers contribute. Fully realized, participatory research contemplates "researchers and local people work[ing] together as colleagues with different skills to offer, in a process of mutual learning where local people have control over the process."[22] On this model, all should contribute to defining the problem to be studied and to producing, analyzing, presenting, controlling, and using the research findings. In practice, participatory research occurs on a continuum, with local communities exercising varying degrees of authority and involvement.[23]

A look at one study shows how participatory research can work. During the mid-1990s, public health researchers from the University of California joined staff members of a community health center and members of the Korean American community to conduct a project funded by the Centers for Disease Control and Prevention. Researchers chose the topic in consultation with health center staff, which included community members. The plan was to conduct a five-year controlled trial to assess an intervention's effectiveness in improving cancer screening rates among Korean American women. Investigators enlisted a diverse group of community leaders and other residents to serve as advisers and decision makers throughout the study. This group met monthly with the investigators, and decisions were made by consensus. Community members were also hired for several staff positions.

In response to comments from the community advisory group and health center staff, the investigators expanded the study's original telephone survey to address a range of community health concerns, such as violence, race relations, discrimination, stress, and religion. Local community representatives also influenced study methodology, initial study publicity, project interviewer selection, data interpretation, and presentation of study findings. At the insistence of the community health center staff, all study data were kept at the health center, and advisory group consent was required for any future data use.

The project investigators reported that the participatory research approach produced a high survey response rate, more accurate data collection and analysis, and more effective use of survey results. For example, asking questions about religion produced information indicating that outreach efforts should target churches, because a high percentage of Korean Americans participated in church activities.[24]

Participatory researchers and the early HIV/AIDS and breast cancer activists shared similar aims. By the mid-1990s, these aims were accepted in mainstream research settings as well. For example, a 1995 *British Medical Journal* editorial asserted, "patients should help to decide which research is conducted, help to plan the research and interpret the data, and hear the results before anyone else."[25] The same year, an article in *Science* observed, "[p]atients and researchers have different and complementary areas of expertise, and increased patient participation could lead to improvements in the relevance of research questions and in the appropriateness of recommendations arising from studies."[26] And by 1999, officials at the National Institutes of Health (NIH), the major U.S. government funding agency for biomedical research, were urging merit review panels to include more consumer representatives.[27]

Advocacy's Potential Contributions

The material above provides a general sense of the impact advocates can have on research. But what specific contributions can community representatives make? How can individuals who lack formal research training add to a study's quality or make well-reasoned judgments about the merits of different study proposals? Supporters cite scientific, ethical, and practical justifications for community participation.

Enhancing Research Quality

Underlying the campaign for community representation is a concept of research quality that goes beyond its "narrow, technical sense."[28] Enlisting representatives of the study population as members of the research team highlights the moral and social dimensions of the biomedical research enterprise. It acknowledges that this form of research is conducted not simply to answer abstract questions or to satisfy scientific curiosity, but to provide health benefits to society. As analyst Tammy Tengs puts it, "conducting health research is not, of course, an end in itself. Even the knowledge derived from research is not the final product. The real reason to invest in health research is to allay the terror of disease, to prevent it or cure it."[29]

Once one accepts this concept of biomedical research, it is not difficult to envision the ways affected people can help improve research quality. First, members of the community can provide information about which health problems, and which aspects of particular health problems, are most important for scientists to study. Sometimes this will produce surprises. For example, health researchers conducting participatory research on improving health services in Bombay discovered that women in the area ranked better health care below improvements in access to water and electricity.[30] Scientists have devoted relatively little attention to research about treatment side effects, yet almost all people affected by disease want this information.[31] One health researcher predicted that "[g]reater lay involvement in setting the research agenda would almost certainly lead to greater open mindedness about which questions are worth addressing. . . ."[32]

Second, community representatives can provide guidance on how best to investigate a health problem. For instance, when community members were asked their views about a proposed study of aspirin to reduce hypertension in pregnant women, they "asked why there were no plans to follow up the babies of women participating in the trial—[given that] for decades women had been warned not to take aspirin during pregnancy because it might harm their babies."[33]

Third, local knowledge enables community members to spot potential problems with the data that are collected. For instance, in the California cancer screening study described earlier, the project's community advisory group "expressed disbelief at preliminary results showing 'low' overall prevalence for . . . tobacco and alcohol use, actual and threatened violence, and discrimination experiences" and suggested ways to obtain more accurate information.[34]

Fourth, community representatives can help decide whether research results should change clinical practice. For example, after a study showed that large doses of antimalarial drugs during pregnancy could increase infants' birth weights, New Guinea women "living in mud floor huts" pointed out that in their circumstances, bigger babies could make childbirth more risky for both mothers and children.[35] Conversely, when patients perceive research findings as valuable, they want them put into practice. Physicians "might be slow to pick up on the results of important research, but patients alerted to results by active organisations are likely to pay much closer attention and to prompt their doctors to implementation."[36]

Fifth, community representatives can contribute to decisions on research merit. Merit is not simply a matter of elegant design and qualified investigators; it also depends on the social significance of the knowledge a study is expected to yield. Accordingly, the NIH's first merit review criterion is "significance: Does this study address an important problem?"[37] Other merit review criteria, such as innovation, may call for assessment of the potential public health value of a novel research aim.[38] Patient advocates can be as qualified as, and in some cases even more qualified than, researchers to evaluate proposals according to these criteria. Advocates also remind other review panelists "that we don't want simply jewel-like studies that will stay on library shelves but studies that will actually make a difference."[39]

Promoting Ethical Research

Consulting patient and community representatives promotes respect for persons, beneficence, and justice, the basic ethical concepts governing human studies.[40] Researchers convey a message of equality and respect when they honestly seek to discover what matters to prospective study participants and openly admit their uncertainties and concerns about a project.[41] Consulting members of the study population "ensures both that their interests are central to the project or study, and that they will not be treated simply as objects."[42] Such consultation can counter the "experimental colonialism"[43] of researchers who " 'parachuted' in, took samples, and disappeared with nothing of value resulting in the community."[44]

Community representatives can advance more specific ethical objectives, as well. Community members are in a position to know what prospective participants should understand before enrolling in a study.[45] For example, one consumer group considering a model consent form for cancer research asked for "humane and sympathetic" language, risk probability statements, and an emphasis on the voluntary and altruistic elements of study participation.[46] Group members wanted patients to participate in the drafting of forms for specific studies. They called for greater use of methods supplementing written forms, such as videotapes, telephone "hotline" services, and opportunities to talk with people participating in the studies under consideration.

As HIV/AIDS activists demonstrated, advocates can also supply a participant-centered perspective on the potential benefits and harms accompanying study participation. In this way, they can promote defensible decisions on when exposing research participants to risks is justified by a study's expected benefits to participants and future patients.

The concept of community equipoise recognizes this potential contribution. Researchers generally apply the standard of clinical equipoise in deciding when to conduct a clinical trial to compare the effects of different potential treatments. Clinical equipoise exists when there is "honest, professional disagreement among expert clinicians about the preferred treatment."[47] Such disagreement usually rests on experts' differing perceptions of the benefits and harms associated with alternative measures. Because it would be morally indefensible for researchers to give study participants an intervention known to be substandard, genuine uncertainty must exist about which of the potential treatments is better to justify a clinical trial.

But clinical equipoise relies on clinicians and scientists to decide when there is enough uncertainty to warrant a clinical trial. Due in part to HIV/AIDS activists' efforts, support is growing for adopting community equipoise as the relevant standard. According to this standard, a trial should be conducted only if affected people agree with medical experts that there is genuine uncertainty about which intervention is better.[48] Thus, for a trial to be justified, people facing the actual consequences of illness must be uncertain about the preferred approach and want to know which is better. The concept also supports community participation in determining when there is enough uncertainty about the risks and possible benefits of an active agent to justify assigning some participants to a placebo group.[49]

Besides helping to determine when research risks are ethically justified, community representatives can point to risks that might otherwise go unnoticed. For example, through their communications with HIV-positive persons, researchers in the military discovered they needed stronger confidentiality protections for study participants.[50] In another case, a community advisory board supplied guidance on the appropriate financial incentive to offer participants interviewed about attitudes toward HIV and HIV vaccine research. The board pointed out that the incentive should be small enough to discourage intravenous drug users from enrolling to finance their habit.[51]

Community consultation can foster justice in the choice of research participants as well. Distributive justice principles hold that research harms and benefits should be fairly apportioned. Thus, groups and individuals ought not bear a disproportionate share of research risks, nor should they enjoy a disproportionate share of the benefits research produces.[52] Patient and community advocates can help decide whether a proposed study will impose disproportionate burdens on community members or, conversely, will unfairly limit a community's access to research benefits.

Consulting community representatives about the fairness of participant selection can produce varied responses. Disadvantaged communities may seek tangible benefits or control over data in return for their participation. For example, in a Canadian study of HIV/AIDS in six ethnic groups, "[c]ommunity members requested a detailed report of the study results which could be used . . . as a rationale for funding community-based AIDS education initiatives."[53] In another case, the community advisory board for a diabetes project involving Native Mohawks in Canada obtained an agreement giving the community control over study data to prevent "potential misuse of the results."[54]

In contrast, HIV/AIDS activists focused on what they saw as unfair barriers to research participation. In opposing narrow eligibility criteria in clinical trials, they contended that principles of justice supported giving a wider range of people an opportunity to enroll in, and possibly benefit from, trial participation. On a broader level, activists argued that trials with stringent eligibility criteria were unjust because they produced knowledge relevant to only a small percentage of people with HIV/AIDS.[55] These justice-based arguments led to revised participant selection criteria in HIV/AIDS trials and were later invoked by advocates who opposed eligibility criteria that excluded women and disadvantaged populations from research participation.[56]

Incorporating the views of affected persons in research planning and data collection can promote ethical practice in ways that complement and surpass institutional review board (IRB) review. The few members of the general community serving on IRBs cannot be expected to understand the concerns or advocate on behalf of different patient and demographic groups. Even if more community members joined IRBs, the proposal review process could never accommodate the in-depth inquiry necessary for meaningful community involvement. Moreover, the existing ethical and regulatory framework for IRB review fails to incorporate many of the concerns and interests that motivate the advocacy and participatory research movements.[57]

Practical Advantages

As the HIV/AIDS trials illustrated, community involvement can be a practical necessity for research. The reality is that many prospective participants will not enroll if they think researchers have given inadequate consideration to their interests and concerns. This sentiment could become more prevalent if communities gain a better understanding of the uncertainties and risks accompanying study participation. As one HIV/AIDS activist predicted, when well-informed people "are asked to be subjects in a drug trial, increasingly they are going to ask for something more than a sense of moral rightness in return."[58]

Recruitment procedures and materials attuned to local concerns can increase study enrollment. One HIV/AIDS researcher observed that including activists in study planning helped investigators "get a feel for what would play in Peoria. . . ."[59] Investigators in a stroke prevention study commented that voluntary community recruitment counselors were useful in assisting "potential enrollees who might be reluctant or frightened, or . . . undecided about participation."[60] Investigators in Uganda reported that community representatives addressed potential research difficulties related to local politics that would have created "a quagmire for the unwitting outsider."[61]

Community representatives can also alert investigators to problems that could lead participants to withdraw from studies or disregard study requirements during participation. For instance, after a joint meeting on problems in maintaining clinical trial enrollments, investigators and HIV/AIDS activists agreed on several measures (such as permitting people to participate in more than one study at a time) that would make trials more acceptable to participants without undermining scientific standards.[62]

Including community members can produce economic benefits, as well. Although the process of involving community representatives will add to a project's expense, "in the long run the net result will be an improvement in efficiency as a consequence of increased community support, more rapid recruitment, and enhanced cooperation on the part of subjects. . . ."[63] At a broader level, involving community representatives can increase the public's willingness to provide financial support for biomedical research, because many representatives "go back to their own constituencies as allies of scientists rather than critics."[64]

Doubts and Questions

More community involvement could yield an array of improvements in conducting research and applying results. But the endeavor is far from risk-free. Some of the claimed benefits of community involvement merit closer scrutiny. Concern lingers among scientists that lay participation may hinder research progress. Advocates face role conflicts as they attempt to earn the respect of scientists and at the same time maintain credibility with constituents. The move toward community participation raises general issues of justice and fairness as well—who is represented in this process and which interests are advanced?

Are Scientific Quality and Other Research Values Jeopardized?

Though many scientists and clinicians are enthusiastic about community participation, others remain unpersuaded. Community participation challenges traditional notions of research expertise, data ownership conventions, and the professional reward structure. Supporters and opponents disagree on whether there is good reason to alter customary standards and practices in these areas.

Controversy persists over whether laypersons should participate in research merit review. Some researchers contend that consumers on peer review panels are unqualified to judge the caliber of competing proposals. These researchers say that consumers cannot exercise independent judgment in merit review and, as a result, either go along with the majority of scientists on a panel or decide based on considerations not germane to merit. If they side with the majority, consumer panelists "could make it more difficult for creative but unorthodox projects to win funding."[65] If they decide based on external considerations, such as a proposal's "political correctness," they could encourage more funding of "junk science."[66]

At bottom, the controversy over merit review reflects divergent perceptions of research merit. Those who perceive a threat to scientific quality tend to see merit in its more narrow, technical sense. But technical merit is only one component of research excellence. Biomedical research is most valuable when it contributes to important health improvements, and many advocates are fully capable of judging this dimension of research quality. Moreover, the perceived problems with consumer participation are not unique to that group. Scientists on review panels rarely possess expertise in all, or even most, of the content areas of proposals they consider. Thus, they must rely on other scientists to evaluate the quality of those proposals. And even critics of lay participation admit that scientists, at times, evaluate research using inappropriate criteria, thereby preventing meritorious proposals from being funded.[67] Thus, the problems linked to consumer participation already exist to some degree in the conventional approach to peer review.

Another potential threat to scientific and academic values arises when affected communities seek control over research data and the publication of results. Disadvantaged communities most frequently seek this authority, citing past exploitation in research or other social contexts. For example, two primarily Aboriginal communities in British Columbia made control a condition of participating in a diabetes prevention and management project. Health researchers agreed to a set of governing principles that stated that the data "belong to research participants and will be returned to the participants," and "[i]f the community opposes publication of any of the results (data and/or analyses and interpretations), the project team will not publish beyond its reporting requirements to the funding agency."[68]

Such arrangements are novel additions to the biomedical research enterprise. For the community representatives and researchers supporting them, the innovative agreements are a reasonable response to earlier injustices and a morally warranted correction to an unfair convention giving researchers nearly absolute control over data and results. Supporters portray the arrangements as an exercise of the community's rightful authority to protect its members from stigma and other research harms.[69]

Parties to these agreements also believe that the threat to research and academic values is exaggerated. They note that researchers who consult community representatives throughout the study process are unlikely to encounter objections to publication and other desired data uses.[70] One researcher who agreed to a community's demand for prior approval of study publications commented that "[r]eviewers and colleagues shape research," and "[j]ournal editors and publishers influence what topics are published."[71] Why, he asked, should control by community representatives be deemed any more objectionable? Another researcher observed that investigators frequently expect research participants to trust that their interests will be protected. But investigators resist entering into arrangements that require them to trust the community to be reasonable in exercising authority over data use and publication.[72]

On the other side of this debate are scholars and researchers who worry about threats to academic freedom and the integrity of research. An agreement giving a community substantial control over sharing the written products of research "opens up the possibility of serious restrictions on [the researcher's] academic freedom, and encroachment on the academic authority of his . . . university. . . ."[73] Agreements between researchers and study communities could slight the legitimate interests of others with a stake in the project. Researchers receiving financial support to conduct projects usually must promise to share results with the funding source.[74] Researchers may have obligations to report on their projects to employers as well. Their scientific colleagues depend on published findings to guide their own future studies. Most important, censorship of results could impede development of health benefits for the public.

Conflicting obligations to those within the community could arise as well. Which community members should be authorized to control disclosure of research results? What if the choices of the designated community authorities conflict with the preferences of research participants? These broader concerns about the ability and authority of particular individuals to represent group members are discussed below.

Giving the participant community control over data and publication also threatens researchers' personal interests in career advancement, professional prestige, and continued financial support. Control over data and publication are two of many elements of community involvement that can make research more burdensome and less personally rewarding for investigators. Nearly everyone recounting an experience with participatory research warns that it is time-consuming.[75] In the California screening study described earlier, "[u]niversity researchers . . . agonized over prolonged timetables and missed deadlines."[76] Diligence and patience may be needed to engage community members, who typically have many other demands on their time. Involving the community requires "flexibility and a willingness to compromise."[77] At the personal level, it requires "openness, critical self-awareness, iterative learning, humility, patience, respect, and empathy toward the community."[78] Not all researchers will be able or willing to meet these demands.

Research conventions and attitudes create further disincentives. Academic and scientific authorities may label research conducted on the participatory model lacking in rigor and reliability.[79] As a result, researchers may find it more difficult to secure funding for studies or to publish the findings in prestigious journals.[80] Funding agencies may question or forbid community supported deviations from the original research proposal.[81] Agreements to share authorship and other forms of credit with community representatives could be detrimental to an investigator's professional advancement. Professional and institutional adjustments will be necessary for community involvement to gain wide acceptance.

The Politics of Community Representation

Investigators are not the only ones facing new roles in the research process. Community involvement creates new issues for advocates as well. When representatives of an affected community work with investigators to plan, conduct, implement, and evaluate research, they become part of the research enterprise. In the process, they may experience difficulties in maintaining their independence and legitimacy as community representatives.

Advocates may face trade-offs between achieving credibility with scientists and preserving credibility with constituents. HIV/AIDS activists who succeeded in gaining the respect of researchers and government officials underwent a process Epstein calls "expertification."[82] The activists who acquired scientific and medical knowledge about HIV/AIDS came to understand and accept some study requirements they had once opposed. When they began to take the scientists' side on certain research issues, other activists said their former colleagues had become "detached from the[ir] constituencies" and "seduced by the aura of science."[83] Thus, the very achievement that allowed the "expert advocates" to become effective negotiators in disputes over clinical trial requirements threatened their legitimacy as community representatives.

This development highlights the political perils facing advocates who join the research team. If they defend study procedures that other community members reject, they may be accused of co-optation. And co-optation is a real danger, for advocates may be targets for manipulation by others involved in the research process. In California, for example, community meetings ostensibly organized to enable breast cancer activists to discuss possible corporate sponsorship for future studies "became forums in which drug companies instead discussed 'health care reform' and the problems it created for 'industry.'" An activist who criticized this turn of events abandoned her protest after drug company employees threatened to withdraw their financial support.[84]

Community representatives may also be perceived as ineffective. Some researchers and government officials may seek community input primarily for its symbolic or public relations value. In this situation, researchers may pretend to consider community views but proceed to do what they would have done anyway. Community representatives who lack the time and training to monitor studies closely can have a difficult time determining whether researchers have actually responded to their concerns. And if the community opposes what researchers do, or a study has a negative community impact, representatives will be seen as complicit in the objectionable activity.[85]

Finally, advocates and their organizations must make significant time and resource commitments to become active research advisers. Admirers have commented on the "diligent" and "unwavering" devotion of the HIV/AIDS and breast cancer advocates. But they also wonder how long this devotion can be sustained.[86] Exhaustion and cynicism may undermine advocates' commitment, which could in turn undermine the respect they enjoy in the community. Moreover, the organizations they represent may experience internal disputes over whether research advocacy is diverting too large a portion of resources from other parts of their mission.[87]

Authority and Limits of Representation

Communities are not units in themselves, but are made up of different individuals with different values and preferences. What defines a community for the purposes of research design, implementation, and evaluation? What gives someone authority to speak for a community? And what is it that community representatives should represent? How do individuals obtain the knowledge that enables them to act on behalf of others in a group?

Defining a community can pose problems. Often, a community can be defined narrowly or broadly.[88] For instance, in the DOD Program for Breast Cancer Research, two different definitions are used. In first-level peer review, the community is represented by people diagnosed with breast cancer and nominated by an advocacy organization. But in second-level review, the community is represented by an expanded group that includes breast cancer survivors' families, high-risk families, and "others with specific interests and perspectives related to breast cancer."[89] The rationale for using the two definitions is unclear; nevertheless, the approach shows that there are different ways of defining the community affected by breast cancer research.

The diversity of the individuals within a community adds complexity to the task of choosing its representatives. What people outside may see as a well-defined group with a unified outlook can actually be quite heterogeneous:

> The very act of the "community" engaging with outsiders necessitates a simplification of their shared experiences into a form and generality which is intelligible to an outsider. This simplification may imply notions of sameness which border on fictions and often would not pass within the community.[90]

Published accounts of community participation indicate that community leaders or activists usually act as representatives. This makes sense, given that people in these categories "are often the most able to mobilize resources and articulate concerns."[91] The problem is that leaders and activists do not always share the views or interests of other group members.

Leaders may seek to manipulate the research process to increase their personal status and power in the community.[92] Sometimes community power structures exist because certain members of a group unfairly dominate others. By relying solely on community leaders for input, then, researchers can reinforce or exacerbate an unjust situation.[93] For example, few women in developing countries occupy positions of community leadership. As a result, in participatory research involving collaborations with leaders, "knowledge is both provided and produced by men, and women are largely excluded and invisible."[94]

Because activists are often community leaders, relying on them can raise some of the same issues. But choosing activists as representatives also presents distinct issues. Many of the most disadvantaged groups are not served by established advocacy organizations. If investigators depend solely on activists for input, the concerns and interests of the most disadvantaged communities or segments of the community may be left unrepresented.[95] For example, "[w]hite, middle class women prominent in the breast cancer movement" have lobbied for expanded opportunities to participate in clinical research without addressing the financial barriers facing poor women seeking access to such trials.[96]

Activists and mainstream group members may also have different ideas about what constitutes "good research." In the negotiations over HIV/AIDS clinical trial procedures, activists took more radical positions than others in the gay community. Moreover, activists and gay researchers often took opposing positions on trial issues.[97] In this case, activists neither represented the full range of perspectives of gay men with HIV/AIDS, nor represented women, intravenous drug users, and others in the affected community.

Support for the participatory research model is premised on the belief that representatives have privileged information to contribute. Some of that knowledge typically comes from their personal situations, as in the case of someone diagnosed with a serious illness or a family member of such a person. But community representatives ordinarily are expected to provide more than a purely personal perspective. They are expected to provide insights shared by others in the relevant community. Like researchers and clinicians, advocates may assume that they are aware of and can represent a community's preferences and concerns.[98] Yet personal experience cannot, in itself, confer knowledge of "what it is like" for others in similar situations. Direct and ongoing communication with a reasonable sample of community members is essential to genuine representation.

This communication is particularly important for advocates working intensively in research. As they become expert research advisers, they may move closer to the researchers' worldview.[99] In the process, advocates may lose touch with their constituents and, indeed, with the very worldview that qualifies them to act as community representatives. In acknowledging this possibility, an HIV/AIDS activist said that her ability "to do really good work" depended on continued pressure and criticism from "people who *do not* know what I know . . . who are always coming from that very emotional bottom-line place, to keep reminding me about that place."[100]

A final set of questions addresses the substantive views community representatives bring to the table. As long as representatives adopt a reasonably systematic approach to gathering information from constituents, should their views stand as the most legitimate indication of the affected community's interests? On some matters, perhaps not. As we shall see in chapter 3, advocates sometimes overstate the benefits research can provide to participants and the larger community. Advocacy literature at times implies that clinical research is equivalent to treatment[101] and that it is reasonable to expect research to deliver a cure for the disease of interest.[102]

If community representatives bring these attitudes to their research work, they may support study procedures that fail to give adequate protection to participants' interests. Representatives who overestimate a study's potential benefits to constituents may pay inadequate attention to the risks it poses to research participants.[103] One writer graphically raised this concern in commenting on a community advisory board's role in an HIV/AIDS study. He labeled the board a "temporary enabling institution . . . in the research enterprise" and analogized it to the Tuskegee Institute, which helped legitimize the U.S. Public Health Service's syphilis study so widely condemned today. In his words, "the tacit approval of such an institution does not, by itself, constitute ethical, principled, just, or community-sensitive research practice."[104]

Moreover, community representatives who directly or indirectly endorse research could encourage constituents to have a relaxed attitude about participation. Representatives' approval of a trial could "unduly influence individual[s] invited to enter the trial rather than encouraging them to make an informed decision alone."[105] Representatives may be overprotective, as well. Representatives responding negatively to research perceived as potentially damaging to the community could deprive individual members of the opportunity to choose whether to participate.[106] Communities and their representatives may also have "local biases, beliefs, and prejudices" that ought to be disregarded or remedied in the research process. Investigators concerned about the stigmatizing nature of an HIV/AIDS diagnosis, for example, have chosen against enlisting community members to collect data or perform other study tasks.[107]

Effective and Ethical Community Participation

Although numerous questions linger about its proper scope and application, community involvement seems destined to remain part of the health research landscape. In the coming years, researchers and policy makers are likely to experience heightened pressure to include representatives of affected communities in planning, conducting, applying, and reviewing research. But effective and ethical use of this approach will require systematic attention to its practical dimensions and unresolved conflicts of values.

Planning and procedures are crucial. Like other research strategies, the appropriate use of community representation will vary from study to study. As a group of British researchers pointed out, "[i]t is unlikely that there will prove to be one single 'best' approach, but some combinations of types of laypeople and ways of identifying and incorporating their views seem better than others in contributing to particular stages of research."[108] The group urged researchers to plan for community involvement by addressing three general questions.[109]

First, researchers should consider why community advice is desirable for a specific research activity and at what stages the advice will be most valuable. Establishing clear goals and expectations gives direction to community representatives and reduces time spent on extraneous matters. Confronting these questions early allows investigators to design projects that are sufficiently flexible to accommodate revisions based on community reactions. Such planning also allows researchers to allocate the resources necessary to support the desired level of community involvement, including fair compensation for the time and effort of lay representatives. Though some representatives prefer to donate their time, compensation is often necessary to prevent community involvement from becoming a vehicle for exploitation.

Second, researchers should consider who is most qualified to supply the relevant community perspectives. Which groups should participate and how many representatives are needed?[110] To date, the literature on community involvement is largely silent on how researchers and advocacy organizations choose representatives to act on behalf of the affected community.[111] Both researchers and advocacy organizations have responsibilities to include representatives of the primary subgroups that make up a community affected by the research in question. If several advocacy groups serve people with a specific disease or health need, investigators should include representatives from as many groups as is reasonably possible. This is especially important if groups have different positions on community interests relevant to the research.

Third, researchers should consider which methods will best elicit community views. Community meetings and focus groups are suitable for some projects; other situations call for hiring community members as research staff or appointing a community advisory board. Investigators should work with community representatives to develop strategies for communicating with constituents about ongoing research and obtaining information from constituents unrepresented in past advocacy activities.[112]

Descriptions of participatory research highlight a fourth consideration, the educational needs of people involved in a project. To be effective, community representatives often need some understanding of science and the research process. Without adequate training, representatives are likely to become frustrated and cynical about researchers' motives for including them. As the HIV/ AIDS and breast cancer advocates demonstrated, some groups are able to acquire the necessary education on their own. Others will need help with this task, however. Unless the costs of adequate training are built into research budgets, effective community participation will be denied to the most disadvantaged members of society.

Education is needed for researchers as well. Researchers engaged in participatory research often remark on how little their training prepared them for this form of study. It appears that researchers and agencies often see community involvement as a simple adjustment, easily tacked on to the "real" research project. This attitude diminishes the significance and complexity of a truly participatory approach. As the material in this chapter indicates, community involvement presents difficult challenges that require extensive thought and preparation on the part of investigators. Health researchers need formal training to meet these challenges.[113]

Besides addressing these practical elements of the participatory approach, researchers and communities also must attend to its moral and policy dimensions. As we have seen, some researchers fear that consumers engaged in proposal review will compromise traditional standards of research merit. To date, however, no solid evidence exists to support this belief. The mission of the DOD Program for Breast Cancer Research, established in part by consumer representatives, is to fund innovative ideas. This suggests that scientists may have exaggerated fears about lay attitudes toward scientific creativity.[114] Officials from the DOD and other agencies that include consumers on merit review panels report that consumers "usually vote with the scientists."[115] If this observation is accurate, then fears about greater support for "junk science" are exaggerated.

Consumer participation in merit review is a relatively new development, and concerns about its negative impact on science remain speculative at this point. Moreover, it is supported by scientists and government officials with experience on mixed panels. At this stage, the most reasonable approach would seem to be to include consumers in merit review, monitor decisions made by the mixed panels, and examine whether these decisions differ (in positive or negative ways) from those made by merit review panels composed solely of researchers.[116]

Agreements giving communities control over research data and results should receive further scrutiny, as well. Scientific and scholarly freedom, societal interests in publicizing research results, and community interests in avoiding stigma and other research harms are all significant moral considerations. Although it will rarely be appropriate for researchers to grant communities complete control over data and results, the possibility of shared control ought not be rejected outright. Reasonable compromise may be attainable. For example, one Canadian project's agreement provides for power sharing among three partners—a community advisory board, community-based researchers, and academic researchers. Disagreements about data interpretation or communication of research results are to be resolved according to the following terms:

> No partner can veto a communication. In the case of disagreement, the partner who disagrees must be invited to communicate their own interpretation of the same data as an addition to the main communication, be it oral or written. All partners agree to withhold any information if the alternative interpretation cannot be added and distributed at the same time, provid[ed] the disagreeing partners do not unduly delay the distribution of results.[117]

Researchers, advocacy organizations, and funding agencies should evaluate this and other past agreements to develop models for future provisions addressing control over research data and results.

Last, the ethical dimensions of community representation require ongoing attention and analysis. Although representation can enhance the ethics of health research, it is not a panacea. Community representation increases the possibility that the interests of research participants will be recognized and addressed. It is not, however, a mechanism for disentangling all ethical dilemmas that arise in research involving humans. Thus, it should stand as a complement, not an alternative, to other components of research ethics review.

Moreover, community representation comes with its own ethical issues. Attempts may be made to divert representatives from advocacy for community interests to advocacy for an investigator's or research sponsor's interests. Ethical concerns are raised, for example, when community members are enlisted as recruitment counselors to work with frightened or uncertain individuals invited to enroll in research. Representatives who fail to maintain their allegiance to constituents could end up providing "ethical" cover for questionable research practices.

Community representation in the research process is an exciting and promising, but relatively new, development. As the work continues, community representatives, researchers, and scholars should take time to review and reflect on their efforts. Both good and bad experiences should be documented and shared, with the goal of improving the quality of future projects.[118] Investigators and community members alike must be willing to take a hard look at the moral dimensions of their research activities.

As advocates and other community representatives gain power in planning, conducting, and evaluating human studies, they also gain responsibilities to exercise this power appropriately. These responsibilities exist, as well, when advocates and other community representatives participate in decision making at the policy level. In the next four chapters, I examine the moral dimensions of community participation in establishing and implementing policies in three different areas—patients' access to experimental interventions, allocation of funds for research, and protection of research participants.

3

HOPE VERSUS HYPOTHESIS TESTING: EXPANDED ACCESS TO EXPERIMENTAL INTERVENTIONS

[L]ife is composed of specifics. In the short term, we're dead;
the drugs promised for tomorrow are meaningless for those living in hell today. Or such is the view of many PWAs and HIV-
positive people I know. Myself included.[1]

The news that cardiovascular disease is the leading cause of
death among women has been so prominently publicized recently that researchers are occasionally asked to explain this apparent epidemic. In fact, cardiovascular disease has been the
leading cause of death among women for many decades but is
only now being carefully described and studied.[2]

Welcome to NIH's "one-stop shopping" area for information
about clinical trials.[3]

Modern research advocates got their start battling regulations that restricted access to promising experimental interventions. Beginning in the 1980s, activists sought to expand patients' opportunities to benefit from biomedical research. Advocates thought research policies focused too much on avoiding risks to research participants and the public and too little on promoting research benefits. The rules seemed to impede unnecessarily the development of scientific knowledge and new treatments to aid people in desperate need. Advocates targeted government policies for change and in the process helped construct a research system that places high priority on access.

Advocates enthusiastically support government policies that expand access to experimental interventions. Advocates contend that investigational agents and procedures offer people fighting serious illness renewed hope when standard therapies have failed. They also contend that involving more people in research is essential to delivering better therapies to the patients of tomorrow. In Senate testimony, prostate cancer survivor and activist Michael Milken expressed the advocacy community's strong desire for expanded research opportunities:

> If we have a real war on cancer, then why not issue "cancer war bonds"? Why not extend patent lives, accelerate FDA approvals and authorize direct contracting with corporations for research and development? That kind of public–private partnership helped win World War II and it can win World War Cancer.[4]

If constituent benefits were to be measured solely in terms of expanded access, advocates could rightfully claim to have served their constituents well. The picture is more complicated than that, however. Policies hastening drug approval and making investigational drugs available before approval allow seriously ill people to try promising agents when standard treatments fall short. Yet, this approach also has its costs—both to patients using such agents and to others in the community in need of improved treatments. Requirements for clinical research to include more people from previously underrepresented groups could lead to better medical care for group members. Yet patients lacking access to health care will be unable to benefit from the treatments developed through such research. Widespread publicity about opportunities to enroll in clinical trials means that patients have more freedom to participate in the latest research on their conditions. Yet "shopping" for clinical trials requires a savvy consumer.

The campaign for expanded access to clinical research and unapproved interventions blurs the boundary between research and treatment. The campaign encourages patients and the general public to equate investigational interventions with proven therapies. Expanded access can promote this therapeutic misconception at both the individual and collective levels, yielding disappointment, disillusionment, and wasted resources. Responsible advocacy requires tempering enthusiasm for expanded access with a realistic understanding of what investigational interventions can offer study participants and other patients.

The Path to Expanded Access

During the 1980s, advocates for people with HIV/AIDS mounted a vigorous attack on the rules governing access to unproven interventions. Faced with a lethal epidemic and no effective treatments, activists were intensely committed to the search for new drugs to reduce death and suffering. As they embarked on this urgent mission, however, they collided with a drug development system that was slow, inflexible, and highly risk-averse. People with no time to spare were shocked to learn that it took about ten years for new drugs and other medical products to undergo the human testing that was a prerequisite to approval for clinical use.[5]

Displaying banners proclaiming "Red Tape Is Killing Us" and "Release the Drugs *Now*,"[6] HIV/AIDS activists took to the streets and conference halls to protest Food and Drug Administration (FDA) rules on drug testing. With these actions, they joined drug manufacturers and conservative policy groups already lobbying the agency to loosen its approach.[7] By becoming part of this unusual coalition, activists helped set in motion four FDA actions making experimental agents more available to people with HIV/AIDS and other serious illnesses.

One FDA policy change explicitly recognized and amplified a previously informal practice called "compassionate use."[8] The Treatment Investigational New Drug (IND) program, adopted in 1987, allows drug companies to provide study drugs to patients who do not meet formal entry criteria for participation in clinical trials. The program makes available promising, but still unproven, agents to patients with "immediately life-threatening or severely debilitating" conditions who cannot benefit from standard therapies.[9] In 1992, the FDA adopted the parallel track mechanism, which makes new agents targeted at HIV/AIDS available even earlier in the investigational process, as soon as initial safety testing reveals no obvious risks. This program was primarily designed for people with HIV/AIDS who cannot participate in clinical trials for medical reasons or because they are unable to travel to research facilities.[10]

The FDA adopted two additional measures to hasten the approval process for drugs aimed at life-threatening or severely debilitating illnesses. First, in

1988, the agency adopted regulations designed to expedite drug development. The regulations encourage manufacturers to work with FDA officials early in the drug development process so that studies can be designed to generate data sufficient to support approval at a relatively early point.[11]

Another FDA initiative came in 1992. This was the accelerated approval rule, which allows the FDA to rely on so-called surrogate endpoint data in approving new drugs for serious diseases.[12] Before then, drug manufacturers seeking FDA approval had to show that an investigational agent safely and effectively produced "a clinically meaningful endpoint that is a direct measure of how a patient feels, functions, or survives."[13] But waiting for clinical end-point data slowed the study process. For example, an HIV/AIDS drug study had to continue long enough to allow researchers to assess whether the new agent postponed death or prevented opportunistic infections. Activists and community physicians argued that earlier indicators of improvement, such as cell counts associated with stronger immune system function, could be sub-stituted for clinical endpoints. The FDA accepted this argument when it adopted the accelerated approval rule, which permits approval if the experi-mental agent is safe and effective in producing surrogate endpoints reasonably linked with actual clinical improvement.

Although the driving force for FDA action was the HIV/AIDS emergency, the new policy measures had a much wider impact. They produced, for ex-ample, broader and quicker access to investigational agents targeted at cancer, Alzheimer's disease, Parkinson's disease, multiple sclerosis,[14] and heart dis-ease.[15] Because of these revisions, seriously ill individuals unable to benefit from available treatments enjoy increased liberty to seek help from promising but not fully tested interventions.

Activists were also key figures in producing a second set of policy changes that expanded access to experimental interventions. In this instance, women's health advocates were at the forefront in persuading members of Congress and federal agency officials to change the way people were chosen to partic-ipate in clinical research.

This set of developments started in the mid-1980s when a government task force reported that a "historical lack of research focus on women's health concerns has compromised the quality of health information available to women as well as the health care they receive."[16] The National Institutes of Health (NIH) then recommended that researchers seeking federal support include more women as study participants.[17] Five years later, however, a con-gressional review found that the NIH had neither publicized the recommen-dations nor monitored research grants to detect whether more women were included. The reviewers also reported that certain large and expensive NIH studies had enrolled only male participants.[18]

This time, political figures and the popular media paid attention to the findings. By the early 1990s, HIV/AIDS activism had made the public more aware of the personal and social benefits stemming from research participation. There were more women scientists and physicians to speak out against the situation. There were women in Congress to demand meaningful change. There was a woman NIH director, Bernadine Healy, who had the power to make research on women's health an agency priority. Thus, advocates who criticized the omission of women from biomedical investigations had an audience with enough authority and prestige to institute remedial action.[19]

Two major policy changes emerged. In 1993, the FDA abandoned its rule against including "women of childbearing potential" as participants in early phases of drug testing. Officials said studying a new agent's effects in both sexes was needed so that any sex-related differences could be identified early and adequately studied in later phases of clinical trials.[20]

The same year, Congress passed legislation directing NIH officials to ensure that women and members of minority groups were included in government funded studies. In response, officials established guidelines to promote gender and ethnic diversity in study populations. The guidelines instructed researchers to collect data that would allow valid analyses of possible gender and ethnic differences in responses to experimental interventions. The guidelines encouraged research teams to create "appropriate and culturally sensitive outreach programs" to promote study enrollment by people from previously excluded groups.[21]

All these changes in government policy were not without their opponents, for reasons discussed below. Despite the opposition, momentum to expand access to research gathered strength during the 1990s. By the end of the decade, the FDA and NIH were requiring researchers and drug manufacturers to conduct more studies to address children's health issues,[22] and the FDA was requesting more data on how investigational agents affect elderly persons.[23] The overall policy goal was to ensure that all groups shared in the medical benefits produced through research.

After putting in place numerous regulatory revisions promoting access, Congress and agency officials turned to two remaining barriers to research participation. One such barrier was created by patients' lack of awareness of the clinical trials option. Physicians do not always discuss the possibility of trial enrollment with patients, and patients are unlikely to learn about trials from other sources. As a result, patients who might choose to enter a trial are denied the opportunity to do so.[24]

To address this situation, Congress passed a law directing health officials to establish a public database containing information about government and privately sponsored clinical trials of "experimental treatments for serious and life-threatening diseases and conditions." Members of Congress wanted the database to supply the information "in a form that can readily be understood by members of the public."[25] Agency employees charged with developing the database sought advice from patient advocates, who asked that it be made "as broad and as comprehensive as possible."[26] What emerged was an NIH Web page with links to sites describing studies on a variety of health problems and telling visitors how to pursue their interest in enrolling in specific trials.

Financial barriers to research participation were the second target of government action. During the 1990s, health insurers seeking to contain costs increasingly restricted payments for the care of patients enrolled in clinical trials. Research grants typically cover the costs associated with collecting data and providing investigational agents and procedures. But grants ordinarily do not include money to cover hospitalization and other costs of routine patient care for people enrolled in studies. More insurers became unwilling to pay for such care, on the grounds that trial participants received interventions not established as safe and effective. Insurers claimed that covering such interventions would waste resources and raise insurance premiums, which would be unfair to other people in their health plans.[27]

At the behest of advocacy groups and researchers, NIH officials commenced negotiations with managed care plans and other insurers in an effort to expand reimbursement for heath care services to clinical trial participants.[28] Bills mandating coverage for trial participants were introduced in Congress and state legislatures, and some states enacted laws requiring coverage.[29] By 2000, President Clinton had directed the Medicare program to cover routine patient care costs for Medicare beneficiaries enrolled in clinical trials.[30] The measures' supporters argued that health care costs for trial participants were comparable to those for patients not enrolled in trials.[31] They also contended that health insurers had a responsibility to contribute to clinical research that could improve future patient care and help research participants as well. This responsibility was especially strong, they noted, when standard care for serious conditions was either unsatisfactory or nonexistent. Finally, they pointed out that insurers could avoid wasting resources by limiting coverage to trials that had undergone rigorous peer review and were likely to provide important information about potential treatments.[32]

Activists were enthusiastic partners in the campaign to publicize clinical trial availability and increase insurance coverage for trial participants. These programs were consistent with the advocacy view that "increasing patient participation in research . . . is the only means to test newer and better treatments, and thus, save lives."[33] Expanded access has become a motto for advocates, researchers, and federal officials. But it is not clear that advocates should be entirely happy with the consequences.

Access Policies: The Underlying Trade-Offs

Advocates were strikingly successful in promoting policies that made it easier for constituents to obtain experimental interventions through research participation or outside the confines of a clinical trial. They were also successful in persuading government officials to reduce information and monetary barriers to research participation. What accounts for these victories?

Research ethics principles are part of the explanation. Expanded access policies are justified by traditional ethical principles governing biomedical research. At the same time, these principles support constraints on access to protect other important values, such as the welfare of research participants and patients in the community. Moreover, expanded access policies advance less lofty aims. For example, drug manufacturers have been ardent promoters of expanded access. Two analysts once observed that "large parts of the AIDS advocates' critique of the FDA could well have been scripted by the Pharmaceutical Manufacturers' Association."[34] Mixed motives underlie support for programs that promote clinical trial enrollment and make unproven interventions more widely available. An examination of the relevant ethical considerations suggests that advocates would be wise to proceed with care in pursuing the goal of expanded access.

Justifications for Expanded Access

In campaigning for expanded access, advocates could cite three established research ethics principles to support their position.[35] The first was respect for individual autonomy in choices about whether to undergo experimental interventions. In their push for revised FDA drug testing policies, activists contended that people affected by HIV/AIDS were fully capable of deciding for themselves whether to try promising agents before final FDA approval. Advocates argued that restrictive drug testing policies improperly interfered with constituents' freedom to accept possible harm from exposure to unapproved agents in exchange for a chance to improve or extend their lives. The FDA's emphasis on protecting people from the risks of taking drugs that remained under study constituted unjustified paternalism, they charged, particularly in light of the inevitable harm facing people denied an opportunity to try investigational drugs. Under the circumstances, activists claimed, people with HIV/AIDS had little to lose from trying unproven agents.[36]

Later, expanded access proponents continued to raise the autonomy claim. Even after the FDA revised its drug testing policies, advocates accused the agency of violating the seriously ill person's right to choose unproven agents. Senator Connie Mack's 1995 statements are representative:

Before my brother died of cancer in 1979, I found it incredible that he was not allowed to take experimental pharmaceuticals because of a concern over the side effects. It made no sense that while he was dying, faceless bureaucrats in Washington worried about the side effects of a pharmaceutical drug. Terminally ill Americans should be allowed to assume risks with experimental pharmaceutical drugs, especially when there is nothing to lose and may be everything to gain.[37]

In their drive to remove barriers to women's participation in research, women's health advocates also stressed the value of free choice. They argued that exclusionary policies and practices denied women the freedom to decide for themselves whether to enter trials that could improve health care for other women and, possibly, their own care. Advocates claimed such exclusionary policies and practices rested on an outmoded concept of women as helpless and vulnerable creatures unable to make their own decisions. Furthermore, advocates contended, concerns about risks to the children of pregnant study participants were insufficient to justify depriving *all* women of reproductive age of the freedom to choose study participation. Advocates argued that women were not simply "reproductive vessels," they were adults with the same rights to enter studies as anyone else. Accordingly, both women and men considering study participation should be informed of reproductive risks and the importance of contraception in appropriate cases and then be allowed to make their own decisions. [38]

Advocates supporting the two remaining government efforts to expand access also cited patients' freedom of choice as a reason for their support. The government's clinical trials database would give patients coping with illness a wider array of alternatives. Insurance coverage for trial participants would remove financial constraints on patient choice. Together, the programs would advance the goal of making "clinical trials a viable option for all patients."[39]

Activists calling for expanded access appealed to the ethical principle of beneficence as well. They contended that policies limiting access to experimental interventions improperly interpreted the principle's mandate to maximize the benefits and minimize the harms research produces. Restrictions on access had emerged in a different historical context, when the dominant aim was to protect people from unacceptable research harms inflicted earlier in the century. By the 1980s, the research oversight system had been in place for more than a decade and had been reasonably effective in preventing maltreatment of study participants. According to advocates, restrictions on access no longer suited the ethical demands of the times. Now it was necessary, they said, for the balance to shift away from rigid safeguards focused on research risks and toward approaches that could enhance research benefits.

Advocates complained that restrictive policies and practices compromised constituents' abilities to obtain two kinds of research benefits. Activists representing people with HIV/AIDS and other serious conditions stressed the benefits patients could gain through participating in clinical trials or using investigational agents outside a trial. Activists said study interventions often constituted medical treatment for such individuals: "[i]n many instances, the only 'treatment' available to a person with AIDS is within the context of a clinical trial."[40] They also discounted the personal risks of using unproven agents, pointing out that many of their constituents' conditions were inevitably fatal. As one HIV/AIDS activist put it, "[w]e don't know for sure how these drugs will work. But it makes more sense than the next best thing, which is dying without trying anything."[41] Trying experimental interventions offered people with terminal illness a chance of benefit and presented insignificant risk compared to the threat imposed by disease.

Women's health advocates also invoked the beneficence principle in their attack on exclusionary policies and practices. They, too, portrayed the exclusionary approach as an unwarranted bar to seriously ill women's opportunities to benefit personally from research participation.[42] They concentrated even more on a second form of research benefit blocked by the exclusionary approach. The failure to collect adequate data on women deprived women as a class of the medical benefits generated through research. Because women were omitted from studies on HIV/AIDS, heart disease, and other conditions, findings and recommendations did not necessarily apply to them. Ignoring potential sex differences in how people responded to experimental interventions created risks for women who needed medical care or information on prevention strategies. An approach ostensibly designed to allow women to avoid research risks was instead "[p]rotecting us to death."[43]

Advocacy support for government efforts to publicize research enrollment opportunities and secure insurance coverage for clinical trials rested on the beneficence principle as well. Because these programs could trigger higher levels of clinical trial participation, they could hasten development of improved treatments. If more of today's patients enrolled in research, future patients would face fewer health burdens. Measures such as the clinical trials database and insurance coverage for trial participants would lead to better care for the patients to come.

Justice was the third ethical concept cited to support expanded access. The justice principle mandates fair distribution of the burdens and benefits research produces. Once again, advocates charged that exclusionary approaches had become an ineffective way to promote justice in research. Restrictive approaches were a reaction to past research injustices in Nazi Germany and elsewhere. In those cases, scientists had imposed unconscionable burdens on disadvantaged and vulnerable groups to generate knowledge and improved therapies that would help more privileged people. Thus, U.S. government policies were written and interpreted chiefly to prevent disadvantaged groups and individuals from bearing a disproportionate share of research risks.

By the 1980s, however, it was becoming clear that the effort to prevent undue risk had another, less acceptable, consequence. Protecting historically disadvantaged groups from an unfair share of research burdens kept them out of clinical trials that could improve or extend their lives. More broadly, protecting members of such groups from the burdens of research participation meant that study results did not necessarily apply to them. Because of differences in biology and environment, findings from studies conducted on young and middle-aged white men might not generalize to women or to men from different age and ethnic groups. Although people in disadvantaged groups avoided certain burdens when they were omitted from study populations, the omission created burdens in the health care setting, where members of such groups received possibly inappropriate medical advice and treatment based on narrowly focused research.[44] Accordingly, advocates representing women, ethnic minority groups, children, and elderly people called for greater diversity in study populations so that all could obtain a proportionate share of the health benefits research produces.

In sum, advocates championed expanded access as a means of elevating respect for autonomy, beneficence, and justice in biomedical research. Although it is true that expanded access can advance these aims, access alone cannot produce a more ethical research policy. To achieve this broader goal, additional ethical considerations must be taken into account. Moreover, the costs of expanded access must be acknowledged and minimized. A more nuanced understanding of respect for autonomy, beneficence, and justice will assist advocates in developing effective, ethically defensible expanded access programs.

Does Expanded Access Promote Autonomy?

The duty to respect individual choice is one element of the respect-for-persons principle. Respect for persons also incorporates an obligation to protect from harm people who cannot make autonomous choices. Thus, the respect-for-persons principle supports granting only individuals making autonomous decisions the liberty to accept experimental risks.

What makes someone's choice an autonomous one? At a minimum, the person must have a reasonable understanding of the basic information relevant to the choice and be free of undue pressure to decide in a particular way. A person makes an autonomous decision to enroll in a study or try an unproven agent when the decision is adequately informed and voluntary.

The need for adequate understanding underlies the ethical and regulatory requirement that people give informed consent to research participation. The government oversight system requires researchers to describe to prospective participants a study's purpose, the harms and benefits it could produce, and available alternatives to study enrollment. Other study features must be disclosed as well.[45]

Perhaps the most important facts for prospective participants to understand concern the differences between participating in research and receiving treatment in the clinical setting. Clinical care is governed by concern for the patient's well-being; accordingly, such care is specifically designed to meet the individual patient's needs. This patient-centered focus is missing from the research setting. Research projects are designed primarily to produce knowledge; hence, collection of valid data is the primary goal. Study interventions, tests, and other procedures are determined not by participants' individual health needs, but by the study's scientific demands. For example, research participants typically receive fixed doses of investigational drugs, rather than the individualized doses common in clinical care. Also, in many research trials, participants are randomly assigned to receive the experimental intervention, standard treatment, or placebo. Thus, a participant's care is determined by scientific considerations, not by a clinical judgment that an agent or procedure would be best for that particular individual.[46]

Ethicists and policy makers believe it is morally essential for investigators to obtain informed consent from participants before proceeding with research. IRBs spend a great deal of time refining consent forms in an effort to help prospective participants understand important study facts. Despite this commitment to informed choice, empirical evidence suggests that many participants fail to comprehend crucial features of the studies they join.

Evidence of this lack of comprehension comes from studies examining research participants' understanding. Some data come from the Advisory Committee on Human Radiation Experiments, which was established in 1994 to examine unethical research conducted during the Cold War. As part of its work, the committee looked at how participants were faring in contemporary research. In one inquiry, committee staff interviewed 103 patients who had participated in studies. Although most of the patients acknowledged that research is performed primarily to produce knowledge for the benefit of others, many also expressed confidence that clinical researchers would not expose them to any interventions that might harm or fail to benefit them. Some also said they decided to enroll in studies before they were given any information about the risks, possible benefits, and other pertinent facts.[47] Others said they did "not read consent forms carefully because they assume that someone else has scrutinized the risks and benefits on their behalf." These data illustrate "the profound trust participants place in researchers and the research enterprise."[48]

Particularly troubling are data suggesting that cancer patients enrolled in phase I chemotherapy trials have inaccurate impressions of the personal benefits of participation. Experimental drugs and devices ordinarily go through three study phases. In chemotherapy studies, the first phase is designed to discover the maximum dose that people can tolerate. Thus, phase I studies evaluate safety, while later phases explore whether agents are effective against disease. Scientists estimate that only about five percent of participants in phase I trials register a tumor response from investigational agents. Moreover, participants registering a tumor response do not necessarily experience personal benefits in the form of extended or more comfortable lives.[49]

Despite these objective realities, a study involving phase I trial participants found that 85 percent cited as their primary motivation for enrollment the opportunity for therapeutic benefit. Generating knowledge to benefit future patients is, in fact, the major objective of phase I studies. Thus, phase I study participation is fundamentally an altruistic act. But when participants were asked open-ended questions about their primary reasons for enrolling, none mentioned a desire to help future patients.[50]

What accounts for these disturbing findings? Research participants learn about investigational interventions in two settings. One is the research setting, where specific facts about studies are presented. In this setting, the education process has many shortcomings. Consent forms frequently contain language and concepts unfamiliar to the general population. Forms can be so packed with information that it is easy to overlook the most important material. Despite the efforts of IRBs, consent forms sometimes refer to experimental interventions, including placebos and phase I agents, as "treatments."[51] Other terms seem to foster confusion as well. The Advisory Committee on Human Radiation Experiments found that patients' perceptions of potential harms and benefits varied depending on whether a project was called a "medical study" (viewed most positively), a "clinical investigation," "medical research," or a "medical experiment" (viewed least positively).[52]

Besides gleaning study information from consent forms, prospective participants learn through their interactions with members of the research team. But investigators pressed for time may omit the lengthy discussions needed to explain studies to laypersons, or they may impute to listeners a level of understanding that does not exist. Physicians and researchers seeking participants may also present their studies in an overly positive light. A physician discussing this possibility wondered, "[w]hat are physicians involved in clinical cancer research programs *actually* telling their patients about the known or anticipated benefits of experimental therapy? Are they telling them simply to ignore the words 'experimental' or 'of unknown benefit' on the consent forms the patients are required to sign?"[53]

In some cases, researchers themselves harbor unreasonable expectations about the potential benefits of study participation. For example, the study of phase I trials described earlier found that oncologists overestimated the chance that patients would receive health benefits from participation.[54] Unduly

optimistic clinical researchers may pass on their optimism to study participants, who then gain a distorted picture of the research.

For good or ill, people form beliefs about research participation in yet
another setting—that of ordinary life. Popular media reports, study advertisements, and patient advocacy materials shape public impressions of clinical
research. And these information sources frequently overstate research benefits. In the popular media, "[h]ardly a week passes without triumphal news
reports of extraordinary achievement in the laboratory, or of new wonder
drugs."[55] Television and newspaper reports usually describe health research in
a positive light, with few cautions about an innovation's potential dangers or
lack of effectiveness.[56] Advertisements seeking study participants commonly
portray clinical trials as a way for people with medical problems to obtain
therapy. Meanwhile, study risks and placebo control groups are rarely
mentioned.[57]

Advocacy messages paint a similarly rosy picture. Advocacy literature often
refers to investigational agents and procedures as "new treatments" and calls
studies on terminal conditions "life-saving research."[58] The possibility that research interventions might prove ineffective or more risky than standard therapy is seldom broached. Instead, advocates equate clinical trials and medical
treatment. For example, HIV/AIDS activists protested restrictive FDA policies
with the slogan "A Drug Trial Is Health Care Too."[59] In another example,
activists founded the "AIDS Treatment Registry" to distribute to the community information about trials seeking participants. The registry's title implied that trials offered participants proven therapies, "mislead[ing] the community in an important way, engendering in the doing the possibility of false
hope."[60] Similarly, an anthropologist reported that for the breast cancer activists she studied, "[t]he notion of participating in biomedical research was itself
unproblematic. Indeed, receiving experimental therapies through research
procedures was viewed as state of the art care. . . ."[61] Advocates who join researchers and the media in cultivating an image of trials as treatment can
diminish, rather than promote, constituents' abilities to exercise autonomous
choice.

Autonomous choices are both informed and voluntary. Worry about the
voluntariness of patients' decisions to try unproven interventions centers on
two possibilities. One is that people will turn to such interventions out of
desperation to "try anything" to cope with their illness. One physician graphically described how this can happen:

> Incapacitated and hospitalized because of illness, . . . fearful for his health and
> perhaps life, [the patient] is far from exercising a free power of choice when the
> person to whom he anchors all hopes asks, 'Say, you wouldn't mind, would you,

if you joined some of the other patients on this floor and helped us to carry out some very important research we are doing?"[62]

Anguish, fear, and dependence on physicians can drive people to embrace whatever experimental options are offered.

Voluntariness can also be compromised by economic circumstances. A major concern is that people will feel pressured to enroll in research that offers health care services otherwise unavailable to them. This possibility arises because researchers often provide free examinations, health monitoring and education, and study drugs or procedures to participants. These features are especially attractive to people who have no health insurance.[63] In 1999, the *New York Times* reported "[n]obody tracks how many uninsured people seek health care from clinical studies, but researchers agree that they number in the thousands and that their ranks are growing."[64]

Empirical data provide some basis for concern about pressures to enroll. Staff of the Advisory Committee on Human Radiation Experiments interviewed 380 patients who had participated in studies to evaluate potential therapies. Thirty-nine percent said they had had little choice other than to try research participation, presumably because their illnesses were serious and standard treatments had been unsuccessful. Eleven percent said enrollment was the best way for them to "pay" for treatment.[65] Few analysts think that such pressures ought to bar seriously ill and economically disadvantaged people from participating in research. Yet the fact that such pressures exist weakens the argument that expanded access unequivocally promotes individual autonomy.

An emphasis on access to experimental interventions can compromise autonomous decision making in yet another way. Advocates and others who champion expansion of patients' "rights" to try unproven interventions can reinforce reckless and magical thinking among seriously ill patients. People with HIV/AIDS sometimes resort to underground networks to obtain untested agents that later prove toxic and ineffective.[66] Cancer patients sometimes turn to unqualified and often dishonest "healers" in hopes of obtaining miracle cures.[67] It is highly doubtful that people have a realistic picture of the possible harms and benefits entailed in seeking this sort of help. In these situations, unqualified support for access to unproven interventions can promote fraud and exploitation, not respect for autonomy.

Finally, concerns about decisions to try unproven interventions are magnified when expanded access policies target children, dementia patients, and other people who lack the ability to make their own choices about experimental measures. The respect-for-persons principle obligates us to protect vulnerable people from unproven interventions that present unreasonable risk.

Policies to expand pediatric research have the potential to encourage uninformed and desperate parents to enroll their seriously ill children in studies that present significant risks and burdens.[68] Similarly, relatives of dementia patients may harbor unrealistic hope that experimental interventions will restore patients' former abilities or reduce caregiving burdens.[69] Combining expanded access with vulnerable study populations can expose patients to harmful choices by parents and other surrogate decision makers who lack adequate understanding of an investigational intervention's risks and potential benefits and who are reacting to pressures created by patients' ill health.

In sum, expanded access alone will not promote real liberty to choose unproven interventions. True freedom is not advanced when people choose investigational agents or procedures because they have inflated hopes of therapeutic benefit or cannot afford conventional medical care. If informed and voluntary decision making fails to accompany expanded access, respect for persons will be diminished rather than enhanced.

Does Expanded Access Promote Beneficence?

The second major ethical justification for expanded access is its potential to increase the benefits that become available through biomedical research. But the relationship between expanded access and the beneficence principle is far from straightforward. In certain circumstances, expanded access can exacerbate seriously ill patients' burdens and thwart research efforts to evaluate the safety and effectiveness of experimental interventions.

Expanded access offers two kinds of benefits. First, personal gains may accrue to people who enroll in studies or obtain investigational interventions outside trials. Second, expanded access may generate information leading to improved care for future patients. There is no question that expanded access can confer personal benefits, such as extended life, reduced discomfort, satisfaction from actively fighting one's disease, solace in contributing to better care for others, and pride in becoming part of the research "team." As mentioned earlier, study enrollment also can provide participants with certain valued services, such as regular physical examinations and increased interaction with medical professionals.

At the same time, one should not underestimate the possible adverse effects of trying investigational agents and procedures. Study participation exposes people to new risks and burdens. People who try unproven agents outside trials can be harmed in the process. Contrary to Senator Mack's statement, seriously ill and terminally ill patients *do* have something to lose in opting for unproven interventions.

First, some experimental interventions produce side effects that magnify patients' pain and discomfort. Second, though fatalities appear rare, some patients die from the effects of investigational agents or procedures.[70] Third, research participation makes demands on time and energy that could be spent on more pleasant or meaningful projects. Fourth, terminally ill patients who travel to research centers give up opportunities to be with friends and family in their final days. Fifth, terminally ill patients who participate in studies may die in a hospital instead of at home. Sixth, patients trying investigational interventions may be disappointed and depressed when interventions fall short of expectations. Seventh, participants in clinical trials may be disheartened to learn that they received standard treatment or a placebo instead of a promising new intervention. Last, patients and families may assume substantial financial burdens in the form of payments for investigational interventions or research-related procedures.[71]

These possible harms and burdens make expanded access to experimental intervention a mixed blessing for seriously ill persons. It is unclear that trying unproven interventions will do patients more good than harm. Indeed, some analysts express strong doubts that expanded access truly helps patients: "[i]t is not compassionate to hold out false hope to terminally ill patients so that they spend their last dollar on unproven 'remedies' [so] that they might live longer."[72]

Expanded access can also interfere with the production of benefits for future patients. This occurs when expanded access gets in the way of determining whether what appear to be promising interventions actually work. When people can obtain experimental interventions outside the research setting, those intent on trying the latest innovation will be unwilling to enroll in research. Because research participation carries the possibility of being assigned to a control group, patients convinced that a novel approach is their best alternative prefer the certainty of obtaining it outside the trial.[73] Besides creating recruitment problems, expanded access can increase the number of participants who withdraw from trials. Participants who fail to improve during a study may conclude they are receiving standard therapy or a placebo and drop out to seek innovative measures elsewhere.[74]

When expanded access reduces the population of prospective research participants, it can delay or defeat efforts to ascertain whether experimental interventions are safe and effective. In such cases, the future patients who could benefit from such knowledge pay the price of expanded access. Recruitment difficulties and higher dropout rates also increase study costs, reducing the resources available to fund other studies.

These downsides of expanded access are painfully evident in the story of one experimental intervention—high-dose chemotherapy combined with bone marrow transplantation for breast cancer. In the mid-1980s, physicians began administering this procedure to women with advanced breast cancer who had exhausted available treatment options. The procedure had helped patients with other kinds of cancer, and the hope was that it would benefit women with breast cancer as well. The procedure is extremely burdensome and risky. Early on, it caused death in 15–20 percent of the women receiving it, though physicians later were able to reduce the mortality rate substantially.[75] Despite the risks, some women appeared to improve after receiving the procedure. On the basis of case reports and small pilot studies, many physicians, patients, and advocates became enthusiastic about the approach.[76]

By the time it was clear that large clinical trials were needed to compare standard treatment for advanced breast cancer with high-dose chemotherapy and bone marrow transplantation, women were reluctant to enroll. Women willing to take drastic measures to fight their disease found trial participation unattractive, since they might be assigned to the group receiving standard treatment (which had a low success rate). These women instead went to physicians who offered the procedure in the clinical setting. Insurers sought to deny coverage for this costly, unproven intervention, but the denials often were reversed when patients challenged them in court.[77] The upshot was that it took many years for researchers conducting randomized trials to enroll a sufficient number of participants to collect the needed data. Finally, in 2000, several large trials indicated that participants receiving the experimental procedure did no better than those receiving conventional treatment.[78]

In the aftermath of such disappointing findings, some patients and families expressed anger at the physicians and hospitals who provided, and financially profited from, the unproven procedure. In letters to the *New York Times*, two writers said certain breast cancer advocates also were to blame. One writer, whose sister-in-law's transplant "resulted in two anguished months of recovery that might have been spent with her family," wrote: "[b]esides oncologists who are quick to advise untested therapies, we might also reprimand the breast cancer advocate groups who stampeded insurance companies and claimed that life-enhancing therapy was being withheld only because of its cost."[79] The other, a cancer patient herself, criticized the advocates who assumed that anyone questioning the procedure must be "against women's health." From her vantage point as a patient, she wrote, "I want to know that the treatment I receive was developed through solid scientific method, not through flimsy, politically correct ideology and false compassion."[80]

Besides making it more difficult to conduct research, expanded access can lead to premature clinical use of new interventions. The FDA policy on surrogate endpoint data allows drugs to become approved treatments without a clear showing of clinical benefit. In some cases, it turns out that changes in surrogate endpoints are unrelated to actual clinical improvement.[81] Furthermore, because studies using surrogate endpoints are shorter, there is less time in which to detect harmful effects of investigational agents.[82] Thus, as one disenchanted activist noted, "you can have a home-run surrogate marker drug that kills more people than the disease."[83] The FDA makes accelerated approval contingent on a manufacturer's commitment to continue with research that measures clinical endpoints, but the agency has been criticized for failing to enforce the requirement.[84] And even if clinical endpoint data are eventually collected and analyzed, patients can be exposed to harmful and useless interventions during the time between accelerated approval and final data analysis.

These problems led some HIV/AIDS advocates to have second thoughts about accelerated approval. Critics of the approach contend that "it does patients no favor to sell them drugs with serious side effects whose efficacy is unknown."[85] By 1994, these advocates had changed course and were urging the FDA to apply more stringent standards in approving new drugs for HIV/AIDS.[86]

Finally, in evaluating the benefits expanded access offers to future patients, it is important to maintain a balanced perspective on the contributions research can make to improved treatment for serious illness. It is unrealistic to expect research to deliver speedy and comprehensive cures for cancer, Alzheimer's disease, psychiatric disorders, and many of the other diseases that motivate research advocates. Contrary to Michael Milken, more research is unlikely to "win World War Cancer"; rather, it is likely to yield incremental improvements over the years. More achievable are significant advances in treating and preventing infectious diseases such as HIV/AIDS, but in this field, as well, hopes for a "quick fix" often go unfulfilled.

Just as patients ought not enter trials based on inflated expectations of personal benefit, advocates ought not promote expanded access based on inflated expectations of treatment benefits to patients. When advocates seem to promise that speedy cures will emerge if research opportunities are expanded, they can mislead study participants and disappoint other patients awaiting the miracles. Such promises can also lead to a loss of congressional and public support when research fails to deliver the goods.

In sum, efforts to expand access to investigational interventions should rest on well-founded estimates of the possible benefits and harms accompanying such access. Recall that the beneficence principle creates an obligation to maximize the benefits and minimize the harms research produces. Access policies consistent with the beneficence principle will incorporate responsible predictions of their positive and negative impact. Allowing unreasonable hope to shape access policies could diminish the benefits and amplify the harms generated by the research enterprise.

Does Expanded Access Promote Justice?

Advocates for women, ethnic minority groups, children, and elderly people see expanded access as a means to correct an unjust distribution of research benefits. They believe that expanded opportunities for research participation will enable constituents to secure a more fair share of the health improvements research can provide. Many patients and clinicians also see research participation as a matter of justice. Indeed, one article observed, "[w]e have entered an era in the United States in which exclusion from participation in medical research is often viewed as a discriminatory denial of beneficial treatment."[87] Yet close examination suggests that expanded access policies can produce only a limited impact on distribution of health benefits. Broader financial and social inequalities constrain the ability of expanded access to rectify health care injustices.

Expanded access to research and unproven interventions must not be confused with expanded access to health care. First, increased opportunities to enroll in clinical trials can do little to meet the needs of those unable to afford adequate health care coverage. Any personal health benefits people gain through study participation usually end with the study. Second, because the FDA permits drug companies to charge for investigational drugs distributed under early access programs, access can be limited based on patients' ability to pay.[88] Third, accelerated approval of investigational drugs for clinical use offers no help to uninsured patients or those in health plans that fail to cover the new treatments.[89] Activist Larry Kramer commented on the irony of this situation:

> AIDS activists have furiously pressured and battled the research establishment to get new drugs conceived, developed, tested and marketed. So for the first time an awful lot of people who thought they were dying are saying "Maybe we'll live through this plague after all." And an awful lot of people should be thinking, "If I can afford it."[90]

The bottom line is that expanded access to investigational interventions can do little to help uninsured and underinsured study participants and other patients secure meaningful access to the beneficial therapies produced through research.

Similarly, the campaign to secure insurance reimbursement for trial participants' patient care costs overlooks people with no insurance at all. As one writer noted, "[f]or poor women and women of color . . . who currently have difficulty in obtaining coverage for mammography, funding for experimental therapies would be difficult, if not impossible, to locate."[91] Advocates argue that "no one should be excluded from research studies because they cannot afford the standard care costs that are associated with a study"[92] But remedying this injustice leaves intact the more widespread and serious difficulties faced by people who cannot afford standard care *outside* the research context.

Income disparities are also likely to restrict the beneficial impact of increased access to information about clinical trial enrollment. Websites that describe clinical trials will be of no use to people who lack access to the Internet.[93]

Furthermore, income disparities will influence the distribution of health benefits produced by research incorporating diverse study populations. New knowledge about the health needs of women, ethnic minority groups, children, and elderly people will not help those unable to afford the clinic visits, new drugs, or lifestyle changes that could improve their health. At the same time, keeping the commitment to develop such knowledge requires researchers to recruit more members of disadvantaged groups for study participation. Recruitment programs aimed at such groups offer reimbursement for travel, child care, meal, and other expenses associated with study participation.[94] Some studies also provide support groups for patients participating in trials, which "can be very helpful to low-income and elderly populations who do not have the resources to provide support themselves."[95]

The problem with such incentives is that they can induce people to join studies they would refuse if they were financially better-off. A related problem arises when members of disadvantaged groups seek health care through clinical trial participation. If opportunities to enroll in clinical trials increase, and the number of people with adequate health coverage decreases, research will become a more enticing means for low-income people to obtain a modicum of clinical attention. The outcome could be that members of disadvantaged groups end up bearing an undue share of research burdens *and* lacking a fair share of the health benefits produced through research.[96]

A final concern is that patient groups represented by effective advocates will disproportionately benefit from expanded access policies. In the case of the parallel track program, for example, HIV/AIDS activists convinced the FDA to adopt an early access policy that applied solely to their constituents. Some analysts believe that interest group lobbying has influenced FDA decisions granting early access to drugs aimed at other conditions as well.[97] If agencies make decisions about access to experimental interventions in response to advocacy pressures, patient groups represented by skilled advocates are likely to reap an unfair share of the benefits conferred by such access.[98]

It is not surprising that expanded access to experimental interventions can have only a minor effect on distribution of health benefits. Expanded access policies and programs are implemented in a system riddled with economic and social inequalities. Disparities in wealth and education will determine how the benefits and burdens of increased access are distributed. To achieve a more just distribution of research benefits and harms, advocates must press policy makers to address problems in the distribution of health care and other social goods as well.

Toward Ethically Defensible Access Programs

As we have seen, expanded access can have both good and bad consequences. At its best, expanded access can increase individual freedom, enhance research benefits, and produce a more just allocation of research benefits and harms. At its worst, expanded access can foster uninformed decisions to try unproven interventions, hamper efforts to evaluate such interventions, and lead low-income people to join studies in hopes of obtaining a fraction of the health care services they need.

Advocates can play an important role in determining how expanded access turns out. Advocates bring a unique perspective to the search for access programs that appropriately balance different and sometimes competing ethical considerations. Their personal experiences with illness and close contacts with others similarly affected give advocates special knowledge and authority to address the ethical problems raised by expanded access. Many advocates are also well versed in the scientific, clinical, and policy issues relevant to access. This mixed expertise provides a strong foundation for advocates' work on access policies and practices.

At the same time, advocates' intimate familiarity with the experience of illness can make them vulnerable to excessive optimism about what access can offer. Advocates sometimes evaluate expanded access in ways that are "passionate and unreflective, not a result of cool appraisal."[99] Unwarranted confidence in the value of access pervaded the early years of HIV/AIDS activism, when many advocates implied that cures would quickly emerge once investigational agents became widely available. Similarly, some women's health advocates seemed to let wishful thinking color their opinions of high-dose chemotherapy and bone marrow transplantation for breast cancer. Advocates who are themselves fighting disease, and those with loved ones in that position, may find it difficult to face certain cold, hard facts about scientific progress—that it is slow, highly uncertain, and complicated to measure.[100]

Advocates' vulnerability to excessive optimism about the benefits of expanded access is understandable, and perhaps unavoidable. When advocates represent constituents in the policy arena, however, they assume a responsibility to assess access realistically. Prospective research participants are not well served when advocates downplay the risks of trying unproven interventions or imply that access to research is equivalent to access to proven treatment. Patients are not well served when advocates allow expanded access to stymie the research necessary to determine the value of experimental interventions.

Besides their own reluctance to confront the shortcomings of expanded access, advocates may encounter external pressure to portray access as an unmitigated good. Clinical research is in the midst of a growth period. Projects in both the academic and private sectors are greatly in need of research participants. In this climate, drug companies and other research sponsors realize that advocates can be valuable allies in their quest to boost study enrollment.[101] Corporations and professional groups that stand to benefit financially from accelerated approvals and other FDA access decisions know advocacy organizations can advance their cause.[102] Advocates should be attuned to the possibility that research sponsors will attempt to manipulate advocacy activities to further their own agendas.

Once these potential problems are recognized and addressed, advocates can contribute to access policies that give due regard to respect for persons, beneficence, and justice. The first aim is to promote autonomous decision making by constituents exercising their expanded freedom to try experimental interventions. To date, researchers, policymakers, and ethicists have achieved only partial success in helping people understand important facts about research and investigational interventions. Advocates are in a good position to improve this situation.

Some patient advocates have themselves faced choices about whether to enter clinical trials or try unapproved agents outside trials. Most advocates have relatives, friends, and colleagues who have confronted such choices. Advocates' insights into the experience of deciding for or against experimental alternatives can provide the basis for more effective patient and public education about the process.

Certain advocates have already used their knowledge to create model informational materials for people considering participation in cancer[103] and psychiatric research.[104] In communications with constituents and the general public, they have stressed both the altruistic nature of research participation and the differences between participating in research and receiving clinical care.[105] They have discussed the context in which access operates, seeking to enlighten people about matters such as the FDA approval process,[106] probability and risk in research, and why randomization and control groups are important in evaluating new interventions.[107] They have warned constituents of the dangers of trying unapproved agents obtained through underground networks.[108]

Advocates can engage in additional activities to ensure that patients and the public receive accurate information about research. They can notify researchers when advertisements and consent forms make study participation appear more attractive than the facts warrant. They can monitor the government's clinical trials database and seek revisions if the materials put too positive a slant on trial participation. They can voice dissatisfaction with science and media reports that exaggerate the clinical significance of research "breakthroughs."[109] They can support policy initiatives to remedy the tendency of corporate and other research sponsors to publicize only studies whose results favor a new drug or procedure.[110]

Another matter ripe for advocacy attention is the phase I chemotherapy trial. Researchers should frankly acknowledge to patients the low incidence of health benefits to participants in such trials.[111] Patients facing a terminal prognosis are not in the best position to be active and demanding research decision makers, however. Advocates could perform a valued service by helping to develop strategies for delivering the facts about phase I studies in a straightforward yet sensitive manner.

Finally, advocates can send a clear message that their support for expanded access is contingent on preserving patients' rights to adequate information. An example is this statement by the director of a leading mental health advocacy organization:

> Our strong support for research hinges upon the appropriate care of consumers who volunteer as research subjects. Consumers who are considering participation in research, along with their care-giving family members, must be fully aware of what the protocols involve, what risks they face, what options they have, and who they should contact with questions or issues as they arise.[112]

Reminders of the need for informed decision making encourage constituents to demand and consider carefully the important facts about a study or investigational intervention before choosing to go forward. Announcements like this also put researchers and industry sponsors on notice that the advocacy community will not allow enthusiasm for access to overshadow requirements for accurate and effective disclosure.

The second aim is to establish access policies and practices that strike a reasonable and ethically defensible balance between the benefits and harms research can produce. Although advocacy support for expanded access policies remains strong, the emergence of negative consequences has generated reservations as well. When it became clear that investigational agents could be ineffective or dangerous and that access could hinder research to determine which agents were safe and effective, certain HIV/AIDS activists qualified their enthusiasm for expanded access. They openly questioned the benefits of the FDA's accelerated approval program, arguing that patients would be better off if the agency applied more rigorous standards in deciding when new drugs may be marketed for clinical use.[113]

Certain women's health advocates also took strong stands against widespread availability of high-dose chemotherapy and bone marrow transplantation for breast cancer. Fran Visco, president of the National Breast Cancer Coalition, was one. Visco contended that insurance coverage should be available only to women enrolled in studies evaluating the procedure.[114] After the trial data showing no benefit were released, she criticized oncologists for their continued reluctance to oppose clinical use of the procedure. In this situation, Visco insisted, patients would be better served if constraints were placed on their access to a burdensome and questionably effective intervention.[115]

Advocates in touch with the worlds of illness and science are in a good position to help evaluate whether access restrictions reflect unwarranted scientific or bureaucratic conservatism or, alternatively, incorporate well-founded judgments that risks are unreasonable in relation to expected benefits. Moreover, if advocates are included in the evaluation process, the resultant decisions are likely to gain wider public acceptance than are decisions issued by officials and scientists alone.

Advocates who seek to reconcile access and beneficence must have the fortitude to give constituents unwelcome news about innovations billed elsewhere as potential cures for their afflictions. But as Steven Epstein writes, if advocates can cut through the hype surrounding early trials of investigational agents, "and communicate the *relative uncertainty* of such trials to the broader public," patients might be more cautious about trying unproven agents and more accepting of the need for rigorous studies prior to widespread clinical use.[116]

The third challenge is to design and implement access policies that promote just distribution of research burdens and benefits. Requiring more representative study populations is a small step toward ameliorating disparities in access to health benefits. A more significant step would be to ensure that medical advances produced through research are available to all in need. Advocacy organizations that give access to experimental interventions top priority risk neglecting constituents' more basic interests in access to established clinical care. Advocates who concentrate on removing financial and other barriers to clinical trial participation risk overlooking barriers to standard treatment. Constituents are better served when advocacy organizations approach justice from a broad perspective and work for increased access to the benefits available through both established treatments and experimental interventions.[117]

Besides promoting fair access to health care, advocates can promote fair application of policies to expand access to investigational interventions. In this vein, advocates can work to ensure that policies to increase diversity of study populations are maintained without the use of overly appealing incentives for research participation. They can operate outreach programs to supply the Internet services that will allow people to take advantage of the government's clinical trials database. They can encourage sponsors to continue to provide study participants with beneficial experimental agents after studies have ended.[118] Finally, by seeking to improve constituents' access to health care, advocates can lessen the chance that patients will enter studies to obtain services they cannot obtain outside the research setting.

In sum, veracity and a degree of objectivity must go hand in hand with expanded access. Patients and the public must be given an accurate picture of what can be gained and lost through participating in studies and trying unproven interventions. Freedom to choose is important, but so is awareness of what is being chosen. Moreover, the value of expanded access must not be overrated.

Advocates can play key roles in promoting justifiable expanded access programs. They can start by resisting their own temptations to exaggerate the benefits such programs hold for research participants and other patients. They can guard against allowing their desire for better treatments to undermine their responsibility to warn constituents of the risks and uncertainties associated with unproven interventions.

In the public arena, advocates can fight against the common tendency to see major scientific advances as representative of research in general. Advocates can be openly skeptical when researchers, corporate sponsors, and journalists label novel interventions "cures" and "breakthroughs." They can emphasize how often initially promising agents and procedures are later revealed to be more risky or less effective than standard treatments. They can stress the scarcity of "research rescues" and tell the stories of patients whose resort to unproven measures had a less happy ending than those typically recounted.[119]

Though this stark, even pessimistic approach may seem callous, anything less straightforward risks encouraging false hope. Patients are free to maintain unwarranted optimism about their prospects, but the research system is not free to exploit this vulnerability to advance its own ends. Biomedical research is driven in part by the desire to escape our status as mortal biological creatures, a desire often shared by people coping with serious illness.[120] By entering research and obtaining investigational interventions, patients can avoid facing the harsh realities of their situations. But the avoidance is often temporary and can come at great personal cost. Investigational interventions can distract people from care options that offer more comfort and freedom to pursue important personal projects. By keeping patients aware of alternatives to experimental measures, advocates can counter social attitudes that foster unfounded faith in such measures.

Advocacy for expanded access to experimental interventions is one way to promote constituent interests. Yet constituents have a wealth of additional needs and concerns that cry out for advocacy attention. Expanded access programs will almost always make relatively modest contributions to the well-being of current and future patients. An appreciation of the limits of expanded access will supply the strongest ethical basis for research advocacy.

4

FAIRNESS IN ALLOCATING GOVERNMENT RESEARCH FUNDS

Every year, a U.S. congressional subcommittee hears testimony in a place unofficially known as "Mother Teresa's Waiting Room." In April 1999, a reporter described the scene:

> Here, for three days this week and two days next week, the sick and afflicted and their lobbyists are gathering in an annual telethon of sorts: the competition for research financing to cure disease. Hundreds of ailments are represented, from the most common cancer to the rarest genetic disorder. Even erectile dysfunction received a mention.[1]

The demand for time to testify is so high that just one of every three applicants—chosen by lottery—is permitted to appear, and then for only five minutes.

Why the demand? The subcommittee has a sizable role in determining the research budget for the National Institutes of Health (NIH). Increased financial support for biomedical research is a primary advocacy goal, and advocates hope an appearance before the subcommittee will yield more funding for their constituents. Moreover, because the federal government uses tax dollars to support biomedical research, advocates can make a persuasive case that officials have a moral responsibility to distribute research resources fairly and equitably. Legal requirements and political pressures to engage in open deliberation also make federal officials a prime advocacy target.

High-visibility advocacy activities have transformed the research funding climate, and nowhere more so than in the nation's capital. Decisions that were once rather quietly resolved by officials and scientists have become the focus of a very public and, at times, adversarial debate. In large part, this debate concerns whether the federal allocation system produces a fair distribution of the limited funds available for biomedical research.

The federal government is a leading research sponsor, contributing about one-third of the nation's financial support for biomedical research and development. Industry provides just over half the support. The remainder comes from state and local governments and from private foundations and other nonprofit organizations.[2] Congress sends most federal support for biomedical research to the NIH, an agency in the Department of Health and Human Services. About one-quarter of the total goes to other agencies, such as the Veterans Administration and the Department of Defense, for research on health problems relevant to their missions. Because the NIH is the lead

An earlier version of this chapter is published in *Current Legal Issues 3: Law and Medicine*, ed. Michael Freeman and Andrew Lewis (Oxford: Oxford University Press, 2000) 399–419.

agency for federal funding, however, its practices have attracted the most congressional and public attention.

Congress influences allocation of research resources by awarding designated amounts to each of the institutes and centers that constitute the NIH. The amount Congress awards affects how much research is done in different health areas, because each institute and center is dedicated to the study of a specific health condition (e.g., the National Cancer Institute, National Institute of Mental Health), organ system (e.g., the National Eye Institute), or clinical field (e.g., the National Institute of Nursing Research). At times, Congress exercises even more control by directing or strongly encouraging the NIH to devote a certain sum to a particular disease or other health concern—hence, the high demand for time in Mother Teresa's Waiting Room.

Officials at the NIH also have substantial control over the areas and types of research that receive government support. Officials in the different institutes and centers work with the NIH director to determine the appropriate emphasis for their research programs. Researchers and members of other interest groups influence this decision making as well.

For many decades, this process attracted little public notice. During the 1990s, however, research funding decisions gained a higher public profile. Activists from the HIV/AIDS and breast cancer communities drew media attention to the importance of research funding for their causes. When these groups achieved success in their quest for increased funding, advocates representing patients with other health problems and populations with specific health needs adopted their lobbying tactics. Some advocates began to complain that their constituents had been shortchanged in the funding process, and a competitive environment emerged.[3]

Other developments intensified the public focus on research funding. Debate over escalating health care costs led some to question federal spending for biomedical research on the grounds that research too often led to expensive and marginally beneficial medical interventions.[4] Cost-cutting measures by health insurers reduced hospitals' ability to pay for clinical studies, which triggered requests for increased government support for this form of research.[5] Enrolling in clinical trials came to be seen as a means to obtain cutting-edge therapy for medical problems; general demands for more research in specific areas accompanied this new perception of biomedical science.[6]

By 1996, government officials began to respond to the heightened public scrutiny. Congress held hearings on setting priorities for health research.[7] An NIH working group published *Setting Research Priorities at the National Institutes of Health*, which described in ordinary language criteria and procedures for allocating research funds.[8] The Institute of Medicine, a government advisory organization, issued a report on the strengths and weaknesses of NIH priority setting.[9]

Despite all this activity, the debate over priority setting remains unsettled. Mother Teresa's Waiting Room is overcrowded because advocates believe personal pleas are necessary to protect constituents' interests in adequate research funding. Members of Congress seek favored treatment for afflictions that burden their own families and friends. Scientists perceive threats to their autonomy from congressional and public pressure for concrete health care advances.

The controversy illuminates a neglected question in health ethics and policy: What is a just allocation of resources for biomedical research? Although justice in allocating health care resources is extensively discussed, scholars and policy makers have, for the most part, ignored just allocation in the research context. Philosopher Daniel Callahan describes the prevailing attitude as follows: "we like what [the NIH] is doing, we trust its leadership to make good priority decisions, and we see no good reason to shake the faith of the Congress or the general public about the way NIH goes about carrying out its mission."[10] Traditional neglect of this issue may reflect another common attitude, here expressed by law professor Roger Dworkin:

> The questions of how much money to spend on research and what kinds of research to support are, quite properly, political questions. We elect representatives to decide questions that have no inherently right answers, like . . . how much to spend on basic and how much to spend on applied research; and how much to spend on each of an almost infinite number of worthy ends—cure versus prevention, AIDS versus birth defects, and so forth.[11]

But the increasing debate over priority setting for biomedical research signals a change in these attitudes. Moreover, though research priority setting is inevitably a political process, it also presents moral issues and values tradeoffs that should, at a minimum, be openly acknowledged. In this chapter and the next, I examine the government's biomedical research priority-setting system and the pressures for change. This chapter describes the existing system, the justice issues it raises, and potential reforms. The next chapter analyzes the specific problem of incorporating public perspectives into research priority setting and proposes ways to promote informed and deliberative decision making.

Criteria for Research Priority Setting

The federal government's executive and legislative branches are both involved in setting biomedical research priorities. Each year, the president prepares a budget proposal for the NIH based on recommendations from federal officials. Congress considers the proposal and establishes final budgets for the agency's institutes and centers. If members of Congress think the president's budget devotes an inadequate amount to studies on a particular health problem, they exercise their authority to set aside a specific sum for research on that problem (a process called "earmarking"). Sometimes they adopt a less intrusive strategy and simply encourage NIH to give heightened attention to the areas seen as neglected.

Congressional priority setting seems to rely on factors that typically influence the political process, including constituents' personal interests and the economic welfare of the senators' and representatives' home districts. Self-interest may play a role as well. In the late 1980s, for example, "Washington watchers" attributed legislative earmarks for prostate cancer research to "the large number of politically powerful but aging men who were themselves suffering from prostate problems."[12] Observers also claim that "politicians frequently support additional investments in research on a particular disease after a grandchild or spouse has contracted it."[13]

Recognizing their foibles, a number of House and Senate leaders want to discourage specific congressional directives for biomedical research funding. They believe that NIH officials overseeing the institutes and centers are more qualified to determine how much funding should go to each research area. Advocates of reduced congressional interference see increased NIH accountability as an avenue to their goal. The theory is that if NIH officials offer the public better explanations of their funding decisions and more opportunities to participate in priority setting, Congress will face less pressure to intervene from advocates in Mother Teresa's Waiting Room and elsewhere. As a result of this view, NIH priority setting is undergoing close examination.

The NIH relies on a variety of considerations in allocating research funds. According to the NIH document, *Setting Research Priorities*, the agency's resource allocations are shaped by the following criteria: 1) public health needs; 2) scientific merit of research proposals; 3) level of scientific opportunity in various areas (i.e., whether major advances appear imminent); 4) breadth and diversity of topics and approaches ("[b]ecause we cannot predict discoveries or anticipate the opportunities fresh discoveries will produce"); and 5) training and infrastructure necessary to support current and future research demands.[14] These criteria are not ranked in significance.

Setting Research Priorities also elaborates on the first criterion, public health needs. According to the document, the nation's health needs are evaluated in light of the following considerations:

- The number of people who have a particular disease.
- The number of deaths produced by a disease.

- The degree of disability produced by a disease.
- The degree to which a disease cuts short a normal, productive, comfortable lifetime.
- The economic and social costs of a disease.
- The need to act rapidly to control the spread of a disease.[15]

Setting Research Priorities again takes the position that all these considerations are important and does not rank them in significance. The document notes that exclusive reliance on any one consideration would produce dramatically different priorities. For example, "[f]unding according to the number of deaths would neglect chronic diseases that produce long-term disabilities and high costs to society. . . ."[16]

Setting Research Priorities presents explicit criteria that affect NIH priority setting. Priorities may reflect other criteria as well. Former NIH Director Harold Varmus acknowledged that priority setting may be influenced by desires to 1) preserve the nation's leadership position in science, 2) contribute to economic activities in the private sector, and 3) elevate the public image of science.[17]

Research priorities may also incorporate international health considerations. For example, during the 1990s, the NIH supported studies on preventing and treating AIDS, tuberculosis, malaria, and other health threats to people in developing countries. Former Director Varmus endorsed the use of targeted research funding to promote international relations as well:

> I offer as one example the effort that the NIH has made through the National Cancer Institute to promote a Middle East Cancer Consortium. This effort provides one of the few vehicles that allow representatives of the states of the Middle East to sit down at a common table and talk about common interests.[18]

Finally, citing the negative impact of disease on a country's political stability, he noted that U.S. research funding offers a means to improve the political and economic climate in developing nations.[19]

The Priority-Setting Process

The NIH applies its substantive priority-setting criteria in a lengthy and intricate process. After consulting with institute and center directors (who have previously met with scientists and other interest group representatives), the NIH director submits budget recommendations to the president. Once Congress establishes the final budget figures, officials at each of the institutes and centers have primary control over the division of their funds.[20]

Most NIH funds are used to support proposals from scientists working at NIH or academic research institutions. Usually the agency devotes a little more than half its annual research budget to basic research. Basic research investigates fundamental problems in biology potentially relevant to many health conditions. Though it is possible to predict the health applications of basic research, such predictions are inevitably more speculative than predictions about other types of biomedical research. Indeed, in many instances basic research believed relevant to certain health problems led to important advances in understanding and treating entirely different conditions.[21]

The remainder of the research budget supports applied research and development projects with more specific medical or research goals.[22] Again, however, some predictions about the ultimate application of such projects will inevitably be incorrect, because the research idea turns out to be unworkable or relevant to a different application.[23]

Research proposals are selected for funding according to their merit, which is initially assessed by review panels composed of experts in relevant fields. Five criteria affect merit evaluations: 1) the importance of the problem or question the proposal addresses, 2) the level of innovation in the proposed approach, 3) the adequacy of the proposed research methods to investigate the problem, 4) the investigators' qualifications and experience, and 5) the quality of the research environment.

Funding choices are also made by a second group, the advisory council of each NIH institute and center. Advisory councils are usually composed of two-thirds scientist and one-third public members. After consultation with their advisory councils, institute and center directors may fund proposals that received lower initial merit scores if they think the research is unusually promising or fills gaps in their research portfolios.[24]

NIH officials also have mechanisms to guide the types of proposals they receive. Officials participate in conferences to keep abreast of the problems that preoccupy scientists, clinicians, and advocates. Institutes and centers conduct meetings at which researchers, clinicians, and advocates discuss areas they perceive as underfunded. Based on this information, NIH officials decide when affirmative steps are needed to encourage research interest in a particular area. Agency officials may then sponsor conferences or issue requests for proposals in that area. Finally, the NIH director is authorized to use discretionary funds to support studies in areas identified as especially significant.[25]

This process gives scientists who submit and review proposals a substantial role in determining the direction of biomedical research, which in turn affects how the government invests its research dollars. At the same time, the review process gives NIH officials, advocates, and other nonscientists opportunities to promote funding for particular health or scientific areas.

Problems with Priority Setting

With the increased focus on priority setting have come challenges to the NIH system. One common criticism is that the articulated priority-setting criteria are so general that NIH officials have almost total freedom in their allocation choices.[26] As a result, it is claimed, the curiosity and career interests of the agency's scientist–administrators and their academic research colleagues assume the highest priority in funding decisions. For example, at a Senate hearing on setting research priorities, a representative of the Parkinson's Action Network said NIH had adopted a "laissez-faire" approach that allowed scientific imagination to be the dominant force in shaping research.[27] The speaker claimed this approach had led to relatively low levels of funding for Parkinson's disease research, even though such research would merit substantially higher amounts if the formal NIH criteria were strictly applied.

Another common complaint is that the vagueness of the NIH criteria allows officials to direct disproportionately large sums to disorders represented by highly visible and sophisticated advocacy groups.[28] As a congressional analyst reported, critics believe "NIH spending often follows current politics and political correctness" rather than the articulated public health considerations.[29]

Officials at NIH are criticized as well for their disorganized approach to evaluating public health needs.[30] Currently, the agency's evaluations fail to incorporate well-founded information on the health, economic, and social burdens imposed by various diseases and injuries (a concept known among health planners as "disease burden"). Agency data on the amount it spends for research to address specific health problems are also deficient, because the institutes and centers lack a uniform system for classifying research according to disease relevance.[31]

NIH officials concede that weaknesses exist in their public health needs assessments and their data on spending by disease. In 1999 testimony to Congress, former Director Varmus attributed the deficiencies in NIH figures to the absence of a "common or accepted measure for disease burden" and to difficulties inherent in attempting to assign basic research to specific disease categories.[32] But critics suspect that the lack of solid data provides a convenient excuse when officials are charged with failing to allocate sufficient funds to certain health problems. Moreover, though critics acknowledge that it is impossible to know the precise applications of research, they think NIH officials could do a much better job classifying studies according to their potential relevance to particular medical conditions.

Other critics seek more drastic changes in NIH priority setting. For example, analyst Tammy Tengs challenges the agency's current failure to rank its priority-setting criteria. In her view, "Congress and the Administration should revise NIH's mission statement to clarify that its primary goal should be to produce the greatest possible reduction in the future burden of disease and injury."[33] Moreover, Tengs believes that NIH institute and center budgets should be closely tied to the predicted future burden of disease in their mission areas. She also contends that the agency should do more to create scientific opportunity in the most burdensome disease areas by channeling funds to those areas.[34]

Additional criticism comes from Daniel Callahan, who thinks the existing criteria implicitly envision "progress without end in the improvement of health." He would like to see them replaced with more precise and realistic goals, such as "relief of pain, suffering and disability to the level that the majority of those liable to suffer from them are able to function effectively as persons, citizens, and workers."[35] He argues that too heavy an emphasis is placed on research to extend the average life span, and not enough on studies relevant to disease prevention, public health, symptom relief, and amelioration of disabilities.[36]

The other primary target of criticism is the NIH funding process. Most frequently raised are problems with the agency's approach to the public. Many say that the NIH has done a poor job of publicizing opportunities for public participation in priority-setting discussions. Because larger, well-financed advocacy groups are best able to monitor NIH activities, they have been the ones taking advantage of public participation opportunities. As a result, critics contend, these groups have had a disproportionate effect on how research funds are divided.

Finally, patients and their advocates seek a meaningful role in priority setting. As one congressional witness noted, "[s]ome patient groups believe the decisionmaking process at the NIH is basically a closed process where patient organizations are only consulted at the later stages, when decisions in fact have already been made."[37] At another meeting on priority setting, an advocate reported that public participants, "though politely received, often come away feeling patronized."[38]

The debate over NIH priority setting raises questions of distributive and procedural justice. Participants in the funding debate disagree about the appropriate considerations to guide funding choices. They also disagree about the appropriate federal process for research priority setting and the place of the public in that process.

Distributive Justice Considerations

Distributive justice principles seek to determine a fair allocation of benefits and burdens in society. These principles are at the heart of the debate over

NIH priority setting. Because taxpayers bear financial burdens to support government research, officials are obligated to do what they can to ensure that research resources are fairly distributed. The priority-setting debate addresses whether certain health and scientific areas receive disproportionately high levels of funding while other areas receive disproportionately low levels. Of course, what is "disproportionate" depends on one's view of the proper criteria for allocating research funds.

To get a sense of the hard choices faced in funding allocation, consider just a tiny subset of candidates for NIH funding: studies to determine the "late effects" of chemotherapy and radiation in adults who survived osteosarcoma, Hodgkin's disease, and other childhood cancers;[39] research on a vaccine to prevent HIV;[40] studies on the potential connection between childhood cancers and pesticides;[41] research on new diagnostic, preventive, and treatment measures to address the oral health needs of children under five and low-income populations;[42] high-volume sequencing to establish the order of DNA bases in the human genome;[43] outcomes research to assess the effectiveness of different clinical interventions;[44] studies to understand why low-income and certain ethnic groups have higher rates of cancer and lower survival rates;[45] and studies on the incidence and treatment of mental disorders in children and adolescents.[46]

Which of these areas present the most compelling case for federal support? Which present the least compelling? What factors should be considered in making these decisions?

National health needs is one relevant factor. *Setting Research Priorities* lists six criteria for measuring public health needs. They resemble criteria for evaluating where health care dollars are most needed: the degree of harm a condition imposes (in terms of death or disability), the number of persons affected, and the level of associated financial and social costs. Nearly everyone would agree that these considerations are relevant to research priority setting. But as writers who discuss health care priority setting point out, these considerations cannot resolve several significant allocation dilemmas.

One such dilemma concerns the appropriate priority to assign to the "worst off" individuals—those most in need of improved health.[47] This dilemma raises numerous questions in the research funding context. Should the NIH assign highest priority to research on disorders and injuries that cause death or significant disability? When, if ever, should the agency support studies addressing less serious health problems? How should funding be affected by a prediction that significant advances are unlikely in research on a lethal or seriously debilitating disease? What if studies addressing a less serious condition are believed to have a high likelihood of significantly benefiting people at risk for that condition? Finally, the health needs of people in poor countries make them substantially worse off than U.S. residents. Given this disparity, what priority should be given to research on health improvements for U.S. residents as opposed to people in developing nations?

A second unresolved question arises when decision makers must choose between distributing a limited resource to all who might benefit and reserving it for those with the greatest chance of benefit (the "fair chances/best outcomes" problem[48]). In the research funding context, officials dividing funds between basic and applied research confront this question. Basic research offers some possibility of benefit in a wide range of health areas, while applied studies offer a higher possibility of benefit in more limited areas.

The fair chances/best outcome problem also arises when officials consider whether to invest high sums in areas in which significant research advances seem imminent. Such investments reduce the funds available for distribution to other areas, which in turn reduces the opportunities for unexpected advances in lower-priority areas.

A third distributive justice dilemma is posed by the "aggregation problem," which asks, "when do lesser benefits to many outweigh greater benefits to a few?"[49] This problem faces NIH officials choosing between studies investigating less serious but widespread health problems (e.g., research on arthritis) and studies investigating more serious but uncommon conditions (e.g., adrenoleukodystrophy, the rare but lethal genetic disease in the film *Lorenzo's Oil*[50]). The problem also arises when research funds must be divided between studies that could yield small gains in preventing or treating relatively common conditions and studies that could produce greater improvements in preventing or treating less frequently occurring conditions.

A fourth point of contention concerns whether and, if so, in what situations past neglect requires compensatory justice—in other words, an "affirmative action" approach to research funding. In the early 1990s, for example, women's health advocates called for remedial NIH funding to promote the inclusion of women in clinical trials and to support research on health concerns specific to women.[51] The shift in priorities was justified, they argued, by the agency's earlier failure to devote sufficient funds to women's health research. In turn, some commentators disagreed with this position, claiming the data did not establish that women had been underrepresented in clinical studies and that research on diseases affecting primarily women actually received more than its "fair share" of funds.[52]

With respect to these issues, the research priorities debate raises distributive justice problems similar to those encountered in health care priority setting. But certain distributive justice problems are intensified in the research context because of the greater uncertainty characterizing predictions of benefit. This is particularly true with basic research, but the uncertainty exists for applied research and development as well.

Research is necessary because it is unknown whether particular lines of inquiry will lead to health benefits. Initially promising ideas often fall short when they are subjected to rigorous study. In such cases, research funds are not wasted, even though they fail to generate health benefits. Further uncertainty is introduced by the many factors that affect whether research knowledge is later translated into practical health interventions. Research funding decisions ought to rest on evidence-based predictions that a study will produce knowledge relevant to improved health care. But the link between funding and health benefits will always be more tenuous in the research context than it is in decisions on health care priorities.[53]

Resource allocation in the research context is also especially troublesome because it requires numerous trade-offs between benefits to people who will experience the burdens of disease in the near future and people expected to suffer health problems in the more distant future. For example, officials would face such a trade-off in choosing between funding a late-phase clinical trial of a new cancer treatment and funding a gene sequencing project whose health benefits will not materialize for many years. Additional complexity is introduced by foundation and industry funding for research. The presence of other funding sources requires government officials to take into account the private sector's contributions to specific research areas.[54]

Difficulties in Evaluating the Fairness of NIH Allocation: An Illustration

Data from an empirical study of NIH disease-specific funding reveal how morally and practically complicated it is to apply distributive justice criteria to research funding decisions.[55] In the study, health policy analysts looked at the disease burden associated with 29 health conditions. Using six different measures of disease burden, analysts compared the disease burden scores for each of the 29 conditions to the amount the NIH spent for research on those conditions.

For three disease burden measures—the total number of people with the condition, the frequency of new cases, and the number of days people with the condition were hospitalized—the analysts found no relation between severity of disease burden and amount of NIH funding. They found a weak association between level of NIH funding and number of deaths caused by the condition. Funding levels were also weakly associated with years of life lost from the condition. NIH funding was strongly associated with another measure of disease burden known as the disability-adjusted life-year. This measure is based on the number of years of healthy life lost due to disability or death from illness or injury.

The study authors then took the number of deaths caused, years of life lost, and disability-adjusted life-years scores for the 29 conditions and used the figures to estimate the level of research funding specific conditions ought to receive. NIH funds for research on AIDS, breast cancer, dementia, and diabetes exceeded what their disease burdens would justify. Research on other conditions, such as chronic obstructive pulmonary disease, perinatal conditions, and peptic ulcers, was underfunded relative to the burdens these diseases impose. The appropriateness of NIH funding for some conditions varied with the measure of disease burden applied. For example, when number of lives lost or number of years of life lost was applied, NIH funds for schizophrenia and depression research went beyond what the level of burden would justify. But when number of disability-adjusted life-years lost was the basis for evaluating disease burden, these two conditions received less than they should have.

What should we make of these findings? Do they indicate that the NIH distributes its resources unfairly? The findings do raise fairness questions. Why was NIH funding strongly related to only one disease burden measure? Why did perinatal conditions (disorders affecting the very young) and chronic obstructive pulmonary disease (a common and seriously debilitating condition) receive less funding than would be justified by the burdens they impose? Do the findings on AIDS and breast cancer funding verify the claim that NIH officials are too responsive to certain advocacy groups?

It would be a mistake, however, to cite this study as strong evidence of unfair allocation. First, the available data on disease burden have a number of limitations and, as noted earlier, figures on NIH funding by disease are not systematically collected. Second, some of the apparent unfairness may be explained by factors other than disease burden, such as scientific opportunity or past NIH funding levels, "since diseases that have been underfunded in earlier years may deserve additional funding."[56] For example, these factors might justify more funding for studies on AIDS (high scientific opportunity) and breast cancer (prior underfunding). Third, some of the apparently problematic disparities may disappear if the contributions of other funding sources are taken into account. For example, research on pneumonia received less NIH funding than would be justified by disease burden, but this illness is extensively studied by drug companies seeking to develop new antibiotics.[57]

Fourth and most significant, different disease burden measures incorporate different value judgments. Some disease burden measures assume that death and disability at any age are equally important to prevent, some that preventing early death and disability is more important, and some that providing improved quality of life or reduced economic and social costs is as important as preventing death.[58] Thus, one's position on the fairness of NIH allocation will, to some degree, reflect one's position on these values issues.

In sum, like the health care priority-setting debate, the research priority-setting debate cannot be settled solely by reference to distributive justice considerations. Distributive justice analyses can suggest broad, comparatively uncontroversial allocation criteria such as those presented in *Setting Research Priorities*. But these criteria are so general that they leave numerous unresolved dilemmas.[59] An American Medical Association statement on health care priority setting applies equally to the research context: "[d]isagreements about these choices are to be expected because of the diversity of moral, religious, and cultural traditions in this country and the complexity of the task."[60] Similarly, as scholars Norman Daniels and James Sabin observe,

> [t]he weightings that different people give to different moral concerns, such as helping the worst off versus not sacrificing achievable medical benefits, probably depend on how these moral concerns fit between wider moral conceptions people hold. If so, there is good reason to think these disagreements will be a persistent feature of the situation.[61]

According to these and other commentators, the best strategy in such a situation is to create a fair process for making controversial allocation decisions. In the next section, I discuss possible features of such a process.

Procedural Justice Considerations

When modern democracies encounter conflicts in establishing and applying public policies, they look to fair procedures to resolve the disagreements. In the words of Supreme Court Chief Justice William H. Rehnquist, "[a]greed-upon procedures for airing substantive divisions must be the hallmark" of public deliberative bodies.[62] Much of the debate over NIH funding allocation addresses perceived inadequacies in the existing priority-setting process. Empirical and conceptual work on the characteristics of fair allocation systems suggests ways to address these inadequacies.

During the late 1980s, psychologist Tom Tyler conducted an extensive empirical inquiry into public perceptions of procedural justice.[63] Although Tyler's study focused on how fairly citizens thought they had been treated by police officers and judges, he also collected data on and reviewed studies of fairness in other policy contexts, including government distribution of scarce resources. One of Tyler's major findings was that achieving a favorable outcome was *not* the most important factor that affected citizens' evaluations of fairness in official decision making, nor were their evaluations most affected by how much they were able to influence official decisions.

Instead, Tyler found that seven characteristics of official decision making had significant and independent effects on citizens' fairness evaluations: 1) authorities' efforts to be fair; 2) authorities' honesty; 3) authorities' neutrality; 4) authorities' "ethicality"—defined as politeness and concern for citizens' rights; 5) citizens' opportunities for representation; 6) the quality of decisions—defined as whether authorities "had gotten the information they needed to make good decisions" and "had tried to bring the problem into the open so that it could be solved"; and 7) citizens' opportunities to correct errors.[64] Tyler summarized his findings as follows:

> People believe that decisions should be made by neutral, unbiased decision-makers, and they expect the decision-makers to be honest and to make their decisions based on objective information about the issues. . . . People also feel that procedures are fairer when they believe they have had some control in the decision-making procedure. Such control includes having the opportunity to present one's arguments, being listened to, and having one's views considered.[65]

Tyler also determined that most people accepted decisions—even personally unfavorable outcomes—if they were made through a process with these characteristics.[66]

Additional guidance on fairness in research priority setting comes from Norman Daniels and James Sabin, who discuss fair procedures for another kind of priority setting: insurers' decisions whether to cover particular health care interventions. These authors believe that affected persons are more likely to regard decision makers as trustworthy, legitimate, and fair if an allocation system has four features.

First, decisions and their supporting rationales must be publicly accessible. Daniels and Sabin suggest that decision makers develop a written, publicly available "case law" to encourage "more efficient, coherent, and fairer decisions over time, . . . strengthen broader public deliberation and contribute to the perceived legitimacy of the decision-makers."[67] In their view, because the case law approach creates pressure to produce an articulated and thoughtful explanation for a resource allocation choice, the approach will contribute to higher-quality decisions over time.

Second, in a fair allocation system, decisions rest on "reasons those affected by the decisions can recognize as relevant and appropriate for the purpose of justifying decisions to all who are affected by them."[68] Daniels and Sabin think that public articulation of the reasons for allocation decisions can promote a deliberative process in which decision makers and affected persons determine over time what count as acceptable reasons.

Third, a fair allocation system includes a dispute resolution procedure that allows people who "may have been excluded from the decision-making process and whose views may not have been clearly heard or understood find a voice. . . ."[69] According to Daniels and Sabin, such a mechanism will enhance perceptions of fairness and allow decision makers to correct erroneous findings, thus improving the quality of allocation choices. The fourth feature of a fair allocation system is "voluntary or public regulation of the process to ensure that conditions 1–3 are met."[70]

The existing NIH allocation process fails to include many of the features Tyler, Daniels, and Sabin discuss. These omissions may account for some of the controversy over research priority setting. The NIH allocation process could be revised in several ways to take procedural justice features into account.

Devising a Fairer Priority-Setting System

Government priority setting for biomedical research raises difficult distributive and procedural justice issues. Besides presenting controversial values questions, the funding allocation process is complex and multifaceted. Its political and emotional dimensions further complicate the task. Allocation decisions inevitably disadvantage some groups, with serious consequences to them—a classic "tragic choice" situation.[71] Indeed, a desire to keep such painful trade-offs from public view may partially explain the imprecision in NIH priority setting. But the increasingly heated debate over the system's fairness indicates that such an approach is no longer acceptable.[72]

More transparency and accountability are needed to address shortcomings in the current system. As a first step to reform, the existing priority-setting criteria should be reexamined. Reviewers should consider whether to make reduction of disease burden the paramount aim in NIH funding. In such a framework, budgets for the different institutes and centers would reflect the projected burdens imposed by health problems in their mission areas. The remaining NIH criteria (scientific merit, scientific opportunity, breadth of research portfolio, and infrastructure needs) would be applied to determine funding within the different health areas.[73]

Reviewers considering the appropriate role of disease burden in NIH priority setting will be forced to address several controversial issues. They will have to decide whether scientific knowledge should be assigned any value independent of its potential health applications. They will have to consider whether factors such as maintaining international science leadership, elevating the public image of science, enhancing private economic opportunities, and promoting international relations are appropriate objectives for biomedical research funding and, if so, what priority to give to those objectives. They will have to determine what priority to give health research in developing countries, and thus to balance the needs of U.S. residents against the needs of people living in nations unable to support the research.

The inquiry into priority-setting criteria should also explore the values questions implicit in different disease burden measures.[74] The goal should be to establish ethically defensible measures of disease burden for NIH use—most likely, measures that assign significance to the chief elements of poor health: diminished length of life, decreased quality of life, and increased financial and social costs. Reviewers should also consider Callahan's proposal to establish more specific objectives to stand as benchmarks of success in reducing disease burden. Strategies for improving the quality of NIH data on disease burden should be explored as well.[75]

The evaluation of NIH priority-setting criteria should culminate in a revised and enriched version of *Setting Research Priorities*. Unlike the initial version, the revised document should incorporate the views of patient advocates and others not employed by the agency. A draft version should be widely circulated and public comments considered in preparing the final draft.

Congress and NIH officials should use the revised priority-setting document to guide their budget decisions. The revised document should also serve as the basis of a planning system resembling that proposed by Institute of Medicine President Kenneth Shine:

> We ought to hold the scientific leadership of the NIH . . . to a process in which they periodically review their research plans with intramural and extramural scientists as well as other important stakeholders in research and explicitly demonstrate to Congress and the public that they have considered [agreed-upon funding principles] in generating their recommendations to the Congress with regard to the budget. . . . As a corollary to these recommendations, the Congress should hold the leadership of the institutes . . . responsible that the level of research investment in the various disease areas and specific problems is consistent with this set of principles. . . . [76]

Making the agency more accountable to Congress and the public will require changes in traditional NIH practice. The agency's submissions to Congress typically consist of descriptions of research objectives and announcements of research progress. NIH plans and reports should be revised to supply more information about funding allocation. First, plans should set forth the justification for giving high priority to certain research areas and health problems. Second, when scientific opportunity is the claimed reason for assigning higher priority to certain areas, support for this judgment should be provided. Such information is essential to address the suspicion that pure scientific curiosity underlies many funding choices. Third, besides describing high-priority areas, agency plans should disclose areas assigned lower priority and give reasons for the assignment. Retrospective reports on NIH funding awards should disclose which areas received less funding because others were deemed more important to support. When low merit scores on submitted proposals led officials to award a lower-than-expected amount to a high-priority area, reports should include plans for encouraging higher-quality proposals in the future.

Elements of this process should be adopted by officials in individual institutes and centers as well. Institute and center officials should apply the revised NIH priority-setting document to develop specific objectives for research in their mission areas. They should prepare and distribute annual reports that describe how funding decisions advanced their research objectives.

These changes will be resisted by opponents of systematic planning in science. A common refrain is that scientists must have substantial freedom in conducting biomedical research if society is to gain the significant benefits conferred by unexpected discoveries. For medical research, it is often claimed, "the best plan over many decades has been no plan."[77] But the claim that this approach produces greater health gains is speculative. And "serendipity can happen anywhere—including in the context of goal-related research."[78]

Moreover, scientists themselves have questioned the conventional wisdom on research planning. For example, in commenting on resistance to establishing goals and plans for research funding, the editor of the journal *Science* asked, "Does it make sense to be scientific about everything in our universe except the future course of science?"[79]

Similarly, a joint panel of the National Academy of Sciences, National Academy of Engineering, and Institute of Medicine concluded that federal agencies conducting and supporting research can meaningfully evaluate the outcomes of basic and applied research on a yearly basis. The panel rejected the "widespread myth" that the value of basic and other forms of research cannot be assessed in the short term. It also took issue with the claim that science would be harmed by a more systematic approach. The panel instead asserted, "more effective and objective assessments of research programs can only benefit the national research enterprise, both by focusing resources on the most vital fields, and by allocating those resources more effectively."[80]

The changes I endorse would add several fairness elements to NIH funding allocation. Enriched accounts of research plans and actual funding decisions with clear reference to national health needs would give members of the public and their congressional representatives more confidence in the quality of the agency's choices, as well as an opportunity to respond and seek altered decisions in the future. Thus, these documents would perform the case law functions Daniels and Sabin describe. The enhanced disclosure process would also include several of the features Tyler found important to public perceptions of fairness.

Incorporating public perspectives into the priority-setting process is central to these reforms. The reforms contemplate a deliberative process in which government officials, researchers, and members of the public come together both to articulate criteria for setting biomedical research priorities and to struggle with the moral dilemmas and practical complexities of applying those priorities. But incorporating public perspectives into funding decisions presents moral and practical challenges that merit more extensive analysis. The task of constructing a deliberative process in which advocates join traditional participants in research priority setting is the subject of chapter 5.

5

PUBLIC PARTICIPATION IN ALLOCATING GOVERNMENT RESEARCH FUNDS

Almost every major malady has its own laboratory and lobbyist. ... Each malady competes with other maladies for Government money, publicity, and TV movies of the week.[1]

The organizers [of The March—Coming Together to Conquer Cancer] argue that the federal government spends just one penny of every $10 collected in taxes for cancer research. They want more spending on this research, as well as ... the determination by Congress and others that cancer prevention and cure will be top research and treatment priorities.[2]

It's simply a question of whether we're going to meet one of the needs that society has, or whether we're going to meet a number of needs, which would include not only health research, but also strengthening public education, strengthening child care, strengthening job training.[3]

During the 1990s, Congress faced heightened pressure from patient advocates seeking government dollars for studies on specific health problems. Advocates said the intensified congressional lobbying stemmed in part from their dissatisfaction with officials at the lead federal research agency, the National Institutes of Health (NIH). Advocates claimed that though NIH officials gave lip service to the importance of public participation in research priority setting, in reality scientists controlled the agency's funding agenda. Advocates also charged that the agency played favorites, granting overly generous amounts to research on diseases represented by wealthy and politically savvy advocacy groups.

Disturbed by these developments, Congress held hearings on biomedical research priority setting and then asked the Institute of Medicine (IOM), a federal advisory group, "to conduct a comprehensive study of the policies and processes used by NIH to determine funding allocations for biomedical research."[4] In its report, the IOM Committee on the NIH Research Priority-Setting Process urged the agency to expand and formalize opportunities for public participation in funding allocation. By 1999, NIH officials had taken the first steps toward putting this recommendation into effect.

The task will not be simple, however. NIH officials and patient advocates will confront difficult ethical and policy issues as they seek to achieve the goal of increased public participation. For example, if advocacy groups play a more significant role in funding allocation, groups with the resources and expertise to mount the most effective lobbying campaigns could obtain substantial sums for research, while others receive less bountiful amounts. At a broader level, vigorous lobbying for biomedical research funds could persuade Congress to reduce funding for other types of scientific research and other social programs so that the budget for biomedical research can be enlarged. In this chapter, I examine the ethical and policy implications of creating a formal role for patient advocates in research priority setting. I argue that fairness in priority setting will be enhanced if the process is governed by principles of procedural justice and deliberative democracy.

The Emergence of Research Funding Advocacy

Congress is accustomed to interest group lobbying for biomedical research funds. During the 1960s and 1970s, for example, patient advocacy groups

This chapter is a revised version of "Public Advocacy and Allocation of Federal Funds for Biomedical Research," published in *The Milbank Quarterly*, Volume 77, No. 2, 1999. © 1999 Milbank Memorial Fund.

endorsed the establishment of new NIH institutes and centers to focus on specific diseases and conditions. In the past, however, advocacy groups avoided open competition with one another. Although they might work behind the scenes for favorable treatment, the most common public strategy was to endorse general increases in federal support for biomedical research, on the assumption that each patient group would benefit if the country committed more of its tax dollars to research.[5]

By the mid-1990s, however, a new trend had emerged. Although some advocacy organizations still pursued general funding increases, certain disease-specific interest groups took a narrower approach. Citing the success of HIV/AIDS and breast cancer activists in obtaining high levels of targeted research funds, groups representing Parkinson's disease, prostate cancer, and diabetes patients explicitly requested congressionally mandated funds to support their areas of interest.[6] As a representative of the Juvenile Diabetes Foundation International put it, "[t]here was a time when we were very good citizens and really went up to the Hill with one message—overall [funding] for NIH. But it becomes hard as you see other disease areas advance far beyond where we are."[7]

Advocates for diabetes, heart disease, and Parkinson's disease patients also charged that these conditions were unfairly neglected in research funding.[8] In 1996, for example, a reporter wrote that American Heart Association representatives were "complaining publicly that research into heart disease and stroke is being shortchanged compared with research dollars spent per death for AIDS, diabetes, and cancer."[9]

Congress responded to this "threat of siblicide"[10] in a variety of ways. Some senators and representatives supported earmarked funds for specific conditions affecting families, friends, and constituents.[11] Some, including Representatives Ernest Istook and George Nethercutt, sided with the patient groups questioning whether certain conditions, particularly HIV/AIDS, were receiving more than a fair share of the biomedical research budget. These congressmen also challenged NIH officials to explain and defend their funding allocation decisions.[12] In turn, House Appropriations Subcommittee Chair John Porter expressed dismay at the divisiveness. He contended that "the worst thing that could ever happen for biomedical research would be amendments on the floor of the Senate or House that start moving money from one place to another in response to interest groups."[13]

By 1997, congressional concern over increasing competition among disease interest groups led to hearings on biomedical research priority setting.[14] At the hearings, Harold Varmus, the NIH director at the time, described and sought to justify the agency's funding allocation mechanisms. But Myrl Weinberg, representing a consortium of patient advocacy and other health organizations, testified that one reason Congress was experiencing more pressure from disease-specific interest groups was that some felt excluded from the NIH priority-setting process.[15]

After the hearings, Congress sought further information and guidance from the IOM. In 1998, the IOM committee issued its report, *Scientific Opportunities and Public Needs: Improving Priority Setting and Public Input at the National Institutes of Health.* The report expressed support for an increased public role on the following grounds:

> It is clear that broader involvement of the public in discussions about NIH priority setting can result in positive outcomes by enhancing the relevancy of research programs, improving the design and conduct of research, particularly in patient-oriented studies, and assuring all those with an interest in NIH research that there is an opportunity to be heard.[16]

In previous years, NIH officials had made some effort to obtain public perspectives on research priorities. But IOM committee members found that patients and their advocates were not sufficiently represented in NIH priority-setting activities. The committee also observed that the agency's public participation avenues were not sufficiently "user-friendly" to enable all interested groups and individuals to take full advantage of them. In light of these inadequacies, the committee encouraged NIH officials to appoint to their advisory committees more advocates for patients and for special populations, such as specific ethnic groups and traditionally underserved persons.[17]

The IOM committee issued two more recommendations for improving public access to NIH priority-setting activities. First, the committee urged the creation of public liaison offices to communicate with individuals and groups seeking to influence research funding. According to the committee, these offices should be responsible for presenting public views "in a way that can be informative in priority setting" and for documenting NIH responses. The committee also said the liaison offices should develop outreach programs to expand the array of groups and populations able to communicate their priority-setting views.[18]

Second, the committee recommended that the NIH director establish a Council of Public Representatives to help officials 1) increase public participation in and understanding of NIH priority setting, 2) increase and diversify public membership on NIH advisory committees, and 3) take into account the health needs of special populations. This group would also supply "a forum for the director of NIH to interact constructively and in a systematic and regular way with representatives of the public."[19]

In sum, the IOM committee believed that the NIH should respond to congressional concerns about interest group advocacy by establishing more formal and systematic mechanisms to ascertain public preferences on bio-medical research priorities. The committee noted that legislators want to "be able to refer people to an identifiable process at NIH and be assured . . . that the inputs of all interests have been fairly and appropriately taken into account in program and resource allocation decision making."[20] The IOM committee did not supply a detailed description of such a process, however.

Ethical and Policy Implications of Funding Advocacy

What Advocacy Can Offer

It is hardly surprising that people affected by disease and injury seek increased government funding for research on their particular conditions. In this sense, advocacy for research funding is simply an instance of the interest group pol-itics that shape U.S. policy in all areas. People who favor a heightened role for funding advocacy contend that advocacy will produce 1) a research budget more consistent with public preferences and interests, 2) better informed gov-ernment officials and scientists, and 3) medical and psychological benefits for patients and their families.

Patient advocates and their congressional allies claim that NIH officials and scientists have too much authority over the way public funds are spent. The challengers are dissatisfied with the traditional deference NIH decision makers have enjoyed. As Representative Ernest Istook told former NIH Director Har-old Varmus, "[t]he jealousy with which you try to say the pursestrings should be under the control of persons who know better than the rest of us is an attitude that is not healthy in our society, and we are here trying to talk about public health."[21]

The NIH critics suspect that scientists' intellectual curiosity and desires for professional advancement have produced allocation choices that deviate from public preferences and the overall public good. The challengers also suspect that scientists have been overly responsive to certain interest groups, neglect-ing equally deserving but less effective advocates and their constituents. In their view, advocacy already affects NIH allocation; the problem is that not every group has sufficient access to NIH decision makers. Indeed, HIV/ AIDS[22] and breast cancer[23] activists believed their vigorous lobbying was nec-essary to overcome an earlier lack of access to the priority-setting process. From this perspective, creating a more open and inclusive framework for public participation in NIH decision making will yield allocation decisions more consistent with the needs and values of the people whose tax dollars pay for federal research.[24]

Besides producing a more democratic research budget, funding advocacy can augment the information used to generate federal funding decisions. Advocates bring government officials face-to-face with the human costs of an affliction. A graphic account of living with a serious illness or caring for an injured family member conveys personal knowledge missing from the facts and figures Congress and NIH officials ordinarily rely on to make allocation decisions. Advocates also expose NIH scientists to the human side of their work. Besides strengthening scientists' commitment to achieving progress in a particular area, communication with patients and families can lead scientists "to pursue opportunities that might not have been obvious without some knowledge of [the experience of] disease."[25]

Moreover, although channeling money to particular areas cannot, in itself, ensure scientific progress, financial resources are a necessary foundation for such progress. Funds enable scientists to conduct exploratory research, obtain training in previously neglected areas, share ideas, and formulate new avenues for investigation. Advocates seeking increased research funding believe that "[w]ith enough money, [scientific] potential can be created in almost any area."[26]

Patients and their families gain additional benefits from funding advocacy at the federal level. Besides producing increased NIH funding and eventual improvements in treatment and prevention, advocacy can raise public awareness of a condition. Increased awareness can lead to higher rates of state and local funding as well as charitable giving by the general public, wealthy individuals, private foundations, and industry. Lobbying for research funds also can have psychological benefits for patients and families who seek an alternative to passive acceptance of their situations.[27]

Funding Advocacy's Potential Negative Effects

In defending her group's lobbying for research funds, an advocate wrote that a "Capitol Hill swarming with breast and prostate and lung cancer patients, each making his or her case, would seem to be the American way."[28] But in the research funding context, the American way has its pitfalls. Advocates have the potential to enrich the priority-setting process and strengthen the justification for funding allocation decisions. On the other hand, interest group advocacy could contribute to research budgets that 1) exacerbate social inequalities, 2) support poor-quality studies on favored conditions, and 3) neglect other important social programs.

Interest group advocacy for research funds could encourage unfair and inequitable allocations of limited public research dollars. The problems arise because groups with more effective presentations and better access to officials can gain disproportionate advantage over others with less well-financed and savvy advocacy programs. For example, one explanation offered for the lack of research on improving end-of-life care is that "dying patients do not form an energetic, ongoing constituency to advocate for more research," nor do "their survivors [who] tend to be exhausted and grieving."[29]

The trouble with this situation is that the more effective advocates do not always represent the health needs that would be assigned high priority based on criteria such as level of burdens imposed on patients and society or potential for scientific progress. Setting aside funds for research on one health problem often is accompanied by reduced funding for others.[30] If interest group advocacy becomes a more dominant force in research funding allocation, biomedical research could become more concentrated on conditions affecting the rich and powerful. In the meantime, little progress would be made in ameliorating conditions that inflict suffering, disability, and death on disadvantaged people and populations.[31]

Partisan research lobbying could lead to inefficient resource allocation as well. This would occur if powerful interest groups persuaded officials to award funds for research on particular conditions without proper regard for the quality of proposed studies.[32] Poor-quality studies are unlikely to make any contribution to improved health care. Spending money on poorly designed projects in politically favored areas would be wasteful and inconsistent with public preferences and interests.[33]

Last, zealous research advocacy could be detrimental to both constituents and the broader public. Organizations that abandon the quest for increased overall NIH funding in favor of single-interest lobbying risk a loss of influence. As one observer put it, "competition between disease-interest groups has always diluted the research community's ability to 'move the needle' when it comes to funding."[34] And even if the single-interest approach succeeds in the short run, it could endanger long-term funding for research on specific conditions. For example, complaints about disproportionate allocations contributed to an "AIDS Backlash" in Congress and other venues. In this development, patient groups, members of Congress, and media commentators attacked the idea that AIDS is an exceptional illness that merits extraordinary research attention.[35]

Research advocacy also consumes the limited resources of patient advocacy organizations. According to the IOM committee, "interest groups have often produced extensive data sets on disease-specific research spending" to make the case that they receive inadequate funding.[36] More groups reportedly are hiring professionals to lobby for research funding.[37] When advocacy organizations spend substantial amounts to lobby for research funding, rather than for improvements in health care delivery, housing, and other social needs, they arguably compromise their constituents' interests. When organizations focus on increasing funds for research on one condition, they ignore the fact that many of their constituents could be vulnerable to harm from other diseases and injuries.

Zealous research advocacy could have additional detrimental effects on constituents. Vigorous campaigns to promote biomedical research funding could foster unrealistic hope for a "miracle cure" among affected persons and their families.[38] And as an IOM committee on end-of-life care noted, "advocacy groups that champion research to prevent or cure various diseases [often are deflected] from vigorously and publicly promoting palliative research to help those who will, inevitably, die of these causes."[39]

Zealous research advocacy carries potential dangers for the broader public as well. High-profile patient advocacy led Congress to approve significant levels of financial support for biomedical research during the 1990s while permitting declines in support for other areas of research and development.[40] This situation raises questions about the wisdom of investing in biomedical research "at the expense of other vital scientific areas, such as physics, chemistry, energy, and environmental sciences that may be just as worthy as medical research even though they lack its political appeal."[41] Indeed, an overemphasis on biomedical research funding could actually impede advances in biomedical science. As former NIH Director Varmus and others have pointed out, fields such as engineering, mathematics, and physics often yield information that later proves relevant to biomedical research.[42]

Federal tax dollars are also needed to support health care, housing, education, and social welfare programs, many of which assist individuals with health problems. Research funding advocacy could encourage government officials to shift money from these programs to biomedical research, which currently enjoys strong bipartisan support. In 1998 congressional testimony, the chairman of the Indian Health Board voiced this concern:

> Many are excited to hear about President Clinton's new research agenda for the new millenni[um], which is intended to double the budget in the National Institutes of Health to find the cure for cancer. The health research industry, particularly Universities and State Governments, are the winners and the Indian people are the losers who seldom realize any positive gain from this effort.[43]

In sum, research advocacy success could come at the expense of social programs assisting people in need. Ironically, individuals with health problems are among those most likely to benefit from such programs.

A Deliberative Democratic Approach to Funding Allocation

The move to integrate advocates and other public participants into the priority-setting process offers more than a chance to add information and perspectives. Pressure from patient advocates and their congressional allies has compelled NIH officials and advisory groups to take a closer look at the facts and values underlying funding allocation. By putting the spotlight on priority setting, advocates dissatisfied with the traditional process have opened the door to a more thoughtful and systematic approach to allocating biomedical research funds. But what principles should guide priority setting in the future? How can public representatives, NIH officials, and researchers cope with the complicated facts and moral issues relevant to their charge? How can the positive features of public participation be enhanced and the negative features minimized?

Principles of procedural justice and deliberative democracy should govern NIH priority setting. An approach that combines these principles can furnish a realistic and morally defensible foundation for allocating limited research resources in a pluralistic country like the United States. Such an approach is realistic because it acknowledges that members of this diverse society are unlikely to have uniform views on the optimal way to distribute federal research dollars. It is morally defensible because it incorporates basic distributive justice considerations and promotes thorough information gathering, respect for disparate views, reasonable compromise, and ongoing evaluation of decisions over time.

Chapter 4 described conditions ordinary citizens associate with a fair system of allocating limited government resources—conditions such as decision makers' lack of bias, reliance on objective information, and willingness to consider the views of people affected by their decisions.[44] Chapter 4 also discussed characteristics that scholars Norman Daniels and James Sabin consider essential to fair allocation systems, including requirements to explain decisions in writing and opportunities for affected people to correct erroneous findings.[45]

The work of political theorists Amy Gutmann and Dennis Thompson offers additional direction for NIH priority setting. Gutmann and Thompson argue that principles of deliberative democracy should apply in "virtually any setting in which citizens come together on a regular basis to reach collective decisions."[46] They see moral disagreements about allocating scarce resources as prime candidates for a deliberative democratic approach.[47] Indeed, deliberative democracy, as described by Gutmann and Thompson, appears well suited to guide discussions about biomedical research priorities.

Gutmann and Thompson propose three principles to govern deliberative democratic processes. The reciprocity principle requires decision makers to justify their positions by citing reasons that can be accepted by people holding different moral views. The publicity principle requires that the public have access to the facts and reasons justifying a group's ultimate decisions. The principle of accountability holds decision makers responsible for considering the claims of not simply their political constituents but also their "moral constituents," a class that includes all people affected by a group's choices.[48] Gutmann and Thompson also advise that to promote legitimacy in the face of moral disagreement, "deliberative forums should expand to include the voices of as many possible of those now excluded."[49]

Gutmann and Thompson believe that by exposing participants to the claims of a wide range of interest groups, deliberative democracy can discourage bias and divisiveness and promote, instead, a broader conception of the public good. Such exposure can help participants understand the "moral merit" in others' claims, help them see when apparent moral conflicts are actually reconcilable, and allow them to revise over time choices that subsequent deliberation may reveal were unwarranted.[50]

Deliberative democracy, as articulated by Gutmann and Thompson, also includes constraints on democratic choices, constraints imposed by fundamental values. In this way, the approach goes beyond procedural justice principles to guard against the possibility that decision makers will make morally indefensible choices.[51] In the context of allocating research funds, distributive justice principles impose on the government a duty to divide resources in a way that gives individuals a fair opportunity to benefit from federally supported research. This duty can be invoked to rule out extreme positions, such as directing all funds to research concentrated on a single disease, the health problems of one sex or ethnic group, or a single scientific topic.

But as chapter 4 discussed, numerous claims on research resources remain after ruling out all indisputably unfair allocation choices. Deliberative democracy, combined with basic features of procedural justice, supplies a reasonable framework for working out the meaning of fair opportunity in the context of establishing and applying research funding priorities.

An approach that combines deliberative democracy and procedural justice also is more practical and ethically defensible than the available alternatives. In a representative government, advocacy groups are entitled to present their views on the appropriate use of tax dollars to fund biomedical research. As a practical matter, interest group advocacy is likely to persist, even if it is excluded from the government's formal decision-making process. In light of these considerations, the best option is to adopt procedures that give interest groups fair access to the NIH priority-setting process.

Moreover, although opening the door to advocacy participation carries risks, they are not so severe as to justify excluding advocates from the process. Affected groups have a legitimate interest in having their values and preferences represented. In the past, public officials allowed the scientific and medical communities to exercise substantial influence over research funding allocation. Members of these groups are far from disinterested and objective participants; rather, their allocation preferences reflect their personal and professional interests. It would be unfair to deny other interest groups the same opportunity to present their perspectives on funding allocation.

Finally, although problems can arise when advocates are overly partisan, advocates often are more qualified than other members of the public to participate in allocation decisions. Advocates tend to be much more knowledgeable about the personal and scientific dimensions of disease; thus, they are more equipped to contribute to priority-setting discussions. Advocates are also highly motivated to participate. As chapter 6 will show, "neutral" members of the public enlisted to participate in research policy decisions often fail to make meaningful contributions to the process. Advocates have the necessary passion and expertise to add a genuine public voice to research priority setting. Furthermore, an allocation process that incorporates principles of deliberative democracy and procedural justice will encourage advocates to "check their special interests at the door in order to think broadly about science and disease."[52] In the remainder of this chapter, I discuss ways to promote procedural justice and deliberative democracy in research funding allocation.

Designing a Fair Process

The IOM committee recommendations for expanding NIH public communication opportunities are designed to give interest groups fair access to the priority-setting process. The IOM committee urged NIH officials to create a new public advisory committee, make better use of public membership positions on existing NIH committees, and establish public liaison offices. By 1999, NIH officials had responded to the recommendations. The Council of Public Representatives was established and had begun its work.[53] Public liaison offices existed for the director's office and each NIH institute and center, and the NIH Website told visitors how to reach these offices.[54] In a 1999 statement to Congress, then-Director Varmus said that more public representatives would be participating in NIH research planning and review activities.[55]

These actions, although significant, are simply a prelude to achieving deeper and broader public representation. First, to implement the IOM recommendations, NIH officials must devise acceptable selection procedures. There are a huge number of disease-specific interest groups with a stake in NIH participation. They are joined by organizations representing women, African Americans, children, and numerous other populations with interests in certain types of research. As the IOM committee advised, public participants in NIH priority setting should be chosen according to a process that is "fair and perceived to be fair."[56]

So far, the NIH has had mixed success on this front. Before appointing members to the Council of Public Representatives, the NIH director's office issued a call for nominations.[57] Individuals could nominate themselves or someone else. To be eligible, members of the public had to have "special interests" in the NIH, for example, as a patient or family member of a patient; a health care professional; a member of a patient advocacy group; an individual who works as a volunteer in the health field; a scientist or a student of science; a communicator in health, medicine, or science; an individual in public service, academia, or in a professional society touching the medical field.[58]

Nomination letters had to describe the candidate's leadership, communication, and problem-solving skills. Candidates were also evaluated according to their abilities to work effectively in a group, understand and represent "a 'public' view of issues," and "consider broad issues and think 'globally.' " Officials said they would appoint a group with geographic, age, gender, and cultural diversity and with a range of primary interests, including the medically underserved.[59]

This selection process incorporates certain fairness elements but raises two questions. One is whether sufficient efforts were made to encourage nominations from traditionally excluded groups. Although the call for nominations appeared in the *Federal Register* and on the NIH Website, it may not have reached many of the groups the IOM committee described as "unfamiliar with the intricacies of NIH's current complex and varied priority-setting processes."[60]

The decision to include scientists and health professionals on the council raises more substantive concerns. The IOM committee envisioned the council as providing "an organized, regular mechanism for the director to obtain consumer views."[61] But the call for nominations and the initial council appointments expanded the membership to include clinicians and researchers. Among the initial council appointments were three physicians, a nurse, a pharmacist, a speech pathologist, a neuroscientist, a behavioral scientist, and a medical device engineer.[62] With this proportion of traditional experts, it is not clear that the council will supply an authentic consumer perspective.

Conditions for Meaningful Public Participation

Achieving deeper and broader public participation requires more than fair selection procedures. The formal mission of the Council of Public Representatives is to "help bring to the NIH the concerns and interests of the many external publics that have a stake in the agency's activities, programs, policies, and research."[63] The council is also assigned to improve public understanding of the NIH and raise "important matters of public interest" for discussion.

Certain conditions must be met for the council and other NIH advocacy opportunities to amount to more than public relations efforts. A review of the past three decades reveals many instances in which government officials adopted mechanisms for public participation to deflect complaints that experts had too much control over science and technology policy. Often, "[t]he input of public representatives is accepted if it reflects the values that exist within the accepted range of consensus, but is rapidly dismissed as irrelevant or disruptive if it tries to question the boundaries of this consensus."[64]

For the new public participation measures to make a difference, council members and other public representatives must be competent to make meaningful contributions to the funding allocation process. In turn, their contributions must be respected by the officials and researchers accustomed to control over allocation decisions. The success of HIV/AIDS and breast cancer activists in influencing research policy suggests that mutual education is one key to effective public participation.

Chapter 2 described how HIV/AIDS activists gained credibility with scientists and officials by learning enough about the relevant science and medicine to challenge established research approaches. Recognizing that the experience of one's own or a loved one's illness is not enough to create an effective advocate, breast cancer organizations established training programs on science and the NIH system to prepare advocates for participation in research advisory and review groups.[65] Similarly, advocates invited to participate in priority setting will gain more influence if they develop a basic understanding of the NIH and the scientific, policy, and ethical considerations relevant to the allocation process.

NIH officials and the scientists whose work the agency supports must also be open to education. Arrogance and condescension on the part of those traditionally in control of NIH priority setting will doom the effort to incorporate public views. As Richard Sclove observes, injecting democracy into science and technology policy may require "a conscious effort to cultivate mutual respect and trust among collaborating laypeople and technical experts."[66] In the HIV/AIDS negotiations, powerful officials and researchers came to appreciate and value the contributions of informed lay advocates. Similarly, NIH officials and scientists must recognize that public participants possess knowledge that can inform funding allocation decisions.

Officials at the NIH admit that the agency's priority-setting system is imperfect.[67] And in conceding the agency's "need to be more rigorous about priority setting," former Director Varmus wrote that the scientific community must "face the fact that this is a process with subjective components."[68] These are hopeful indicators that at least some officials and scientists recognize that there is room for improvement and that public participants can contribute to a better system for setting research priorities.

Reexamining Advocacy Roles

With advocates' increased abilities to influence priority setting come changed roles and responsibilities. In many NIH activities, advocates will be asked to represent interests beyond those of their customary constituents. They will be asked to represent the general public or a large subset of the population, such as elderly persons, medically underserved communities, or those at risk for genetic diseases. Advocates participating in NIH priority setting must explore and adjust to their new positions. Accompanying their empowerment are new obligations, obligations that for the most part remain to be defined.

In their new positions, advocates will be asked to incorporate a community-based ethic, rather than one based on the interests of a single illness group or population. This task may be less formidable than it initially appears, for a community-based ethic can be consistent with the aim of advancing constituents' interests. Indeed, all interest group advocates should consider the virtues of a more community-based approach.

Advocates should recognize that a single-disease focus could be detrimental to their constituents' interests. As we have seen, competition among interest groups can hamper overall research fund-raising efforts. In the current climate, strategies based on sickness sound bites and dueling diseases seem unlikely to persuade Congress or NIH officials to increase spending for either research on specific diseases or biomedical research in general. Moreover, many constituents will have multiple health needs over the course of their lives; thus, federally funded studies on different health problems could benefit them. Constituents also have loved ones whose health care could be improved by research in a variety of areas. Finally, constituents could benefit from federal support for research in other areas of science and support for social programs, such as health care and housing assistance. Advocates who explore these issues with constituents may find that narrowly targeted lobbying for research funding is inconsistent with constituents' actual preferences.

A strongly partisan approach to research advocacy raises more general moral concerns as well. When advocates lobby Congress and the NIH to obtain the maximum possible research support for their specific constituents, they overlook the compelling needs of other patients. Such disregard for the interests of others is inconsistent with professional and general ethical standards governing advocates' conduct.

Even the pure lobbyist role incorporates responsibilities beyond those owed to constituents. According to the American League of Lobbyists Guidelines for Professional Conduct,

> the professional lobbyist accepts the fact that it is the system of representative government we enjoy that makes possible the practice of lobbying and, while keeping the interest of the employer or client in a position of primacy, will

temper the advocacy role with proper consideration for the general public interest.[69]

Another league guideline directs lobbyists to "acquire enough knowledge of public policy issues to be able to fairly present all points of view."[70] These guidelines would seem to rule out fierce competition by advocates seeking federal funding for specific health problems. The guidelines also create a duty to be sufficiently informed about other biomedical research demands to engage in deliberative discussion of the trade-offs at issue.

Partisan behavior is even less appropriate for advocates representing the public in policy activities related to priority setting. Accordingly, advocates appointed to the NIH Council of Public Representatives should put aside their ordinary focus on specific health problems or populations. Because opportunities to serve on the council are quite limited, it would be patently unfair for the chosen few to concentrate on advancing the interests of specific constituents. NIH officials signaled their agreement with this view by stating that council members must "agree to subordinate disease-specific or program-specific interests to broader, cross-cutting matters of importance to the NIH and its commitment to public representation."[71] Similarly, advocates appointed to institute and center advisory committees should take into account the interests of all groups affected by the particular institute's or center's mission area.

These cautions apply as well to research funding advocates representing scientific, medical, and other professional interest groups. Over the years, advocates for such groups have engaged in extensive lobbying seeking federal research dollars for certain clinical areas or scientific fields.[72] Like patient advocacy, advocacy on behalf of professional groups at times evinces narrow-minded and competitive attitudes. Professionals and their advocates who neglect the broader public interest are just as threatening to fair funding allocation as are narrowly focused patient advocates. Indeed, professionals' expert status and traditional influence over research decision making make them potentially greater impediments to fair resolution of the multiple demands for federal support.

Constructing a Deliberative Process

The hardest task facing all participants is to develop a deliberative democratic approach to NIH priority setting. As chapter 4 pointed out, patient advocates and others involved in the allocation process face numerous ethical dilemmas and practical challenges. Research funding allocation compels decision makers to choose among a multiplicity of health needs and basic science areas that could contribute to improved health. In the background lie broader questions about the proper amounts to budget for biomedical research as opposed to other government programs. Distributive justice considerations offer general guidance on morally appropriate funding choices but fail to resolve several allocation dilemmas.

The situation calls for an ongoing deliberative process in which participants assemble the best available empirical data, explore the range of possible allocation choices, present their positions on the preferred outcomes, and refine those positions in light of what is learned through the process. Successful deliberation will require attention to two major areas.

First, groups engaged in priority setting should incorporate basic elements of procedural fairness. They should develop mechanisms for collecting the views of patient and demographic populations affected by research funding allocation decisions. They should work with NIH public liaison offices to create outreach programs that can counter the access advantages enjoyed by wealthier advocacy organizations. They should prepare written accounts of priority-setting discussions, recommendations, and reasons for recommendations. In these accounts, they should explicitly note which research initiatives were preferred over others, and why. Written recommendations and explanations will allow advocates and others in the community to evaluate the quality of priority-setting recommendations and respond to flaws or errors in the basis for those judgments.

Second, patient advocates, researchers, and other participants will need educational tools to help them cope with the complicated issues and facts relevant to their charge. To fulfill this need, NIH officials should develop materials to assist participants in activities related to priority setting. The materials should be tailored to the particular committee and priority-setting activity in which participants are involved. The goal should be to supply participants with a reasonably accessible account of the considerations relevant to their deliberations.

Some educational materials will be pertinent to most groups' work. As chapter 4 observed, everyone involved in NIH priority setting would benefit from access to good data on public health needs, NIH spending by disease, and biomedical research support from industry and other funding sources.

Participants will also need materials to help them develop more informed and thoughtful views of the priorities and trade-offs they support. Accordingly, groups participating in priority setting could benefit from reviewing past NIH decisions to fund certain research initiatives rather than others and the underlying reasons for those decisions. Another valuable aid to deliberation would be hypothetical cases presenting different options for research funding and delineating the ethical and scientific dimensions of each choice. Through discussing these cases, participants could learn about the multiple factors relevant to research priority setting and the trade-offs that accompany decisions

to invest more in certain research areas than others. The cases could be sup-
plemented with background materials on the potential clinical value of basic
science studies in biology as well as research in other fields.

Reasons for Optimism

In their 1997 report on agency priority setting, NIH officials claimed there is
"no right amount of money, percentage of the budget, or percentage of projects for any disease."[73] But this claim is only partly correct. The "right"
amount or percentage is a function of value judgments on which conditions
merit more research attention than others, together with scientific and practical judgments on where it is realistic to expect progress. The hope is that
increased public participation can yield an expanded and perhaps altered perspective on the relevant facts and values and their relative importance.

Of course, success is far from foreordained. Yet there are reasons to be
optimistic that the deliberative democratic approach will work in research
funding allocation. Although individual advocates, scientists, and officials undoubtedly have different ideas about the best way to allocate funds, most share
a desire to reduce the suffering and death inflicted by illness and injury. Self-
interest and constituent concerns may affect their initial preferences on funding, but most participants begin with altruistic intentions as well. A predisposition to altruism and empathy creates fertile ground for the self-scrutiny
and mutual respect that are essential to successful deliberation.

This predisposition also raises the odds that participants will be open to
learning about the situations and claims of others involved in allocation discussions. Advocates for specific patient groups can recognize that research on
other health problems is a worthwhile cause and may even be important to
their own constituents.[74] Scientists can be reassured that most advocates appreciate the need to maintain basic science research and standards of scientific
quality in the research funding system. Advocates can take heart that the
overriding aim of most researchers and officials is to reduce the burdens borne
by patients and their families.

The increase in interest group advocacy for federal research funds is one
manifestation of advocates' desire to play a greater role in shaping biomedical
research policy. As shown in chapter 3, patient advocates were instrumental
in changing federal policies governing access to unapproved medications and
the age, sex, and ethnicity of clinical research participants. Advocates' participation in priority setting could lead to changes in this area as well. Advocates
have already induced NIH officials to clarify and publicize priority-setting
criteria and procedures. Now officials and advocates face additional challenges
as they attempt to integrate greater public participation with scientific expertise and the government's responsibility to promote the common good.

6

ADVOCATES IN RESEARCH ETHICS OVERSIGHT: A VOICE FOR THE PUBLIC?

═══════════════
═══════════════

The spirit of participatory democracy suggests that the composition of [ethics review] panels should more closely reflect the demographics of the potential pool of [research] subjects.[1]

The goal of including affected populations in research review is laudable, but the likelihood of success in regularly involving a "member of the population being studied" is low.[2]

[C]uriously, the one structure on which activists have focused inadequate attention is the Institutional Review Board. For a number of reasons, this is a logical place for effective and meaningful community input.[3]

At the close of World War II, the Nuremberg Tribunal drew international attention to the dark side of human experimentation. Although the whole world was horrified by the Nazis' blatantly immoral experiments on concentration camp prisoners, two decades would elapse before the United States began to take a hard look at its own research abuses.[4] As people gradually became aware that United States research participants had been exposed to serious risks without their awareness or consent, scientists and government officials faced growing demands for safeguards to prevent similar violations in the future.

Once officials and their advisers went to work on an oversight system to protect research participants' rights and welfare, public representation quickly emerged as a key component of ethics review. Researchers immersed in their projects and culture too easily lost sight of their duty to put research participants' interests above scientific advancement. People from outside the research domain could add an essential moral perspective to judgments about the ethics of proposed human studies.

Public oversight thus became an integral part of U.S. research policy. The Federal Policy for the Protection of Human Subjects assigns primary responsibility for ethics review to research institutions that employ scientists seeking to conduct human studies. Institutional committees formally known as institutional review boards (IRBs) determine whether study proposals meet regulatory and ethical standards for informed consent, a reasonable balance of risks and expected benefits, equitable and fair participant selection, and other participant protections. These committees must include members with no personal ties to the medical school or other facility overseeing the research.

Recommendations to involve the public appear in policies addressing a variety of research ethics issues. U.S. investigators conducting research in developing countries are advised to submit their proposals to ethics review committees that include as members ordinary people living in the community where research will be conducted. Besides serving on review committees, ordinary citizens increasingly participate in other research ethics activities. U.S. rules waiving the customary demands for informed consent in emergency research require scientists to consider the ethical concerns of residents representing the community affected by the research. Researchers conducting studies whose results might lead to discrimination, stigmatization, and related harms to ethnic and social groups are encouraged to seek out and respond to the relevant community's ethical concerns.

Unlike developments described in previous chapters, these initiatives arose without much pressure from patient advocates. In this case, it was primarily government officials, professionals, and scholars who argued for a public role in research decision making. The strongest demand for public involvement came not from grassroots activists, but from "experts" designing the oversight system. What happens to public participation when it originates in official mandates rather than grassroots rebellion? What happens when public representatives are sought out by the powers-that-be instead of admitted in response to advocacy pressure? How might public ethics oversight be altered if advocates devoted more effort to this activity?

This chapter considers patient advocacy in the context of research ethics oversight. Like chapter 2, it examines how advocates can affect the ethics of biomedical studies involving humans. In contrast to chapter 2, however, it analyzes advocates' participation in the specific activity of research ethics oversight, rather than in planning, conducting, and evaluating the merit of research.

The chapter begins with a brief survey of policies calling for public participation in research ethics oversight. I then discuss the aims and shortcomings of public participation in the oversight process. The discussion focuses on public members of IRBs and similar review committees, because such committees are the oldest and most thoroughly examined instance of public ethics oversight. Then I consider what advocates could add to research ethics oversight, describe the possible drawbacks of a more substantial advocacy role, and describe how to minimize the negative effects. I conclude that both ethics oversight and advocacy would benefit if advocates made oversight a higher priority.

Policies on Public Ethics Oversight

Members of the public were not always part of the U.S. research oversight system. The system originated in the 1960s, when officials at the National Institutes of Health (NIH) decided they would require scientists conducting government funded human studies to observe basic standards for informed consent and protection from research risks. The new requirements would be applied by the scientists' "institutional associates." Thus, in its initial guise, ethics review would be performed by a group of the researcher's scientific and medical peers.[5]

A few years later, the rules changed. This time, officials said IRBs should include members competent to judge a proposal's acceptability in light of legal, professional, and *community* standards.[6] Soon after that, the call for members from outside the research establishment was reinforced by the National Commission for the Protection of Human Subjects, a group Congress established to develop ethical principles and guidelines for research. The commission thought that IRBs should be composed of at least one-third nonscientists. Committees with this proportion of nonscientist members would "show awareness and appreciation of various qualities, values, and needs of the diverse elements of the community served by the institution. . . ."[7]

In 1981, the Department of Health and Human Services issued regulations establishing the oversight system that essentially remains in effect today. The regulations, now known as the Common Rule, are applied by most federal agencies that regulate or sponsor human studies. The Common Rule retains the notion that IRBs should include members competent to judge whether research projects will be acceptable to the community. According to the Common Rule, IRBs must have at least five members, including one member "whose primary concerns are in nonscientific areas" and one member with no employment or other close ties to the research institution.[8]

Two additional Common Rule provisions refer indirectly to community oversight and research participant representation. The first provision requires IRBs to have members with sufficient experience, expertise, diversity (in race, gender, and culture), and sensitivity to community attitudes "to promote respect for [the committee's] advice and counsel in safeguarding the rights and welfare of human subjects." The second provision applies to committees that frequently review research involving a particular category of vulnerable participants, such as children or people with mental disabilities. The provision encourages such committees to include as members "individuals who are knowledgeable about and experienced in working with these subjects."[9] Although some people think nonscientist and public IRB members have a special responsibility to protect research participants' interests, the policy itself is silent on this matter. As we shall see, ambivalence about the public's role in ethics review underlies the ambiguous policy references to community oversight and participant representation on IRBs.

After the Common Rule was adopted, U.S. officials continued to endorse public involvement in research ethics review. In a more recent policy development, officials adopted community consultation as a mechanism to reduce ethical qualms raised by waiving the usual demands for participant consent to research. In 1996, the Food and Drug Administration and Department of Health and Human Services issued new rules to govern research conducted in emergency situations.[10] The new rules were triggered by difficulties in testing novel approaches to treating head trauma, stroke, heart attacks, and other emergency health threats.

Applying the ordinary requirement for informed consent to this type of research creates serious impediments to study enrollment because it is often impossible to discuss research participation with people in the midst of a health emergency. By the time a close relative can be asked about the possibility of enrolling an emergency patient in research, it may be too late to try the experimental intervention. The new rules permit research to proceed without a patient's or relative's consent as long as several alternative protective conditions are met. These include a showing that research participants are in a life-threatening condition, no satisfactory proven treatment is available, investigators will allow patients or relatives to make the decision about participation whenever time permits, and animal and other preliminary data suggest the research intervention could benefit participants.

Officials added to these conditions a requirement to publicize study information to the "communities in which the clinical investigation will be conducted and from which the subjects will be drawn."[11] The rules assign to researchers and IRBs a responsibility to consult community representatives about a proposed study and inform the general community about study plans. The idea is to ask community members to stand in for the people who could be enrolled in research without their prior consent and to invite comments about ethical problems a study might pose for emergency patients and their families.

International groups also see community oversight as essential to research ethics review. Most influential in this area are guidelines issued by the Council for International Organizations of Medical Sciences (CIOMS) in collaboration with the World Health Organization.[12] The guidelines focus on research conducted in developing countries, where domestic policy on participant protection can be weak or nonexistent.

Biomedical research in developing countries is often sponsored by agencies and pharmaceutical companies from wealthier nations and conducted by investigators from those nations. In this situation, the possibility of exploitation exists, particularly when the research is relevant to treatment or product development in the richer nation. The CIOMS guidelines establish a system of dual ethics review to prevent researchers and sponsors from taking advantage of economically deprived and poorly educated study participants. Proposed studies must be approved by an ethics review committee in the investigators' own nation and by a committee in the country where the study will be conducted (the "host" country).

The CIOMS guidelines emphasize the need for committees in host countries to include as members "laypersons qualified to represent the cultural and moral values of the community."[13] According to the CIOMS, "the community to be studied should be represented in the review process. . . . It should not be considered that lack of formal education disqualifies community members from joining in constructive discussion on issues relating to the study and application of its findings."[14] Those preparing the guidelines believed that members who understand the local culture are needed to help committees determine the acceptability of proposed methods to elicit participants' informed consent, of any inducements or other benefits offered to participants, and of plans for protecting confidential and sensitive information.

A fourth policy mandate for public oversight may be in the works. In contrast to the previous policy initiatives, community leaders and activists have energetically supported this version of public involvement in research ethics review. In the 1980s and 1990s, the Human Genome Project and other scientific efforts led to a massive increase in genetic research. Some of this research is designed to evaluate genetic variation among human populations around the world. Other studies focus on certain ethnic populations because this makes it easier to trace family histories and identify genetic mutations linked to disease. The hope is that the research will aid in the development of improved prevention and treatment measures that take into account patients' specific genetic characteristics.[15]

Though the research offers legitimate health benefits, it carries risks as well. Leaders of Ashkenazi Jewish, Native American, and other ethnic groups are concerned that genetic research findings could trigger insurance and employment discrimination against people belonging to these groups. Some also fear that their groups will be labeled especially prone to ill health or to specific stigmatizing conditions, such as mental illness or alcoholism.[16] These leaders argue that before going forward, genetic studies should be subjected to ethics review by representatives of the relevant ethnic or indigenous populations.[17]

These are not the only examples of policies and guidelines that endorse public participation in research ethics oversight. U.S. policy requires institutional committees considering the ethics of proposed studies on laboratory animals to have at least one public member who can "provide representation for general community interests in the proper care and treatment of animals."[18] At the national level, nearly all U.S. research ethics advisory bodies have had at least one public member.[19] For example, an executive order required the 18-member National Bioethics Advisory Commission to have at least three members from the general public.[20] Australia, New Zealand, and several European nations have domestic policies calling for public participation in research proposal review[21] and other forms of research ethics deliberations.[22]

Though different in scope and approach, all these rules and recommendations incorporate the judgment that ordinary community residents should have a voice in research ethics review. The official consensus is that members of the general community add a valuable element to research ethics deliberations. But what is that element? Is it more valued in theory and formal policy than in practice? In the next section, I review various justifications offered for enlisting members of the public to participate in decisions about research ethics.

Public Participation Aims

The policies calling for public participation assume that people from outside the scientific and professional realms will enhance research ethics review. In most ethics contexts, however, the public participant's role and responsibilities are unclear. Government officials, commentators, and review committee members make a variety of claims about the benefits of involving the public in research ethics deliberations. Yet many of these alleged benefits are abstract and lack empirical support. It appears that public participation requirements reflect desires not only to make research more ethically acceptable, but also to improve public relations. Moreover, officials seem unwilling to grant the public much real influence over research ethics decisions.

Six Justifications

Surveys of IRB members, together with commentary on the IRB system and other oversight mechanisms, point to six general justifications for including public members. First, public members add a common sense, "ordinary person" worldview that is often missing when professionals discuss research.[23] Public members correct for the myopia that can lead professional groups to accept ideas and practices out-of-step with the broader society. Public members "transform the committee from closed associations of like-minded professionals who 'understand' one another into a more open forum of community responsibility."[24] The unaffiliated IRB member is also free of institutional biases that might distort the ethics review process.[25] Finally, people with no ties to an institution or scientific field are able to discern when researchers and other committee members are guided more by self-interest than by legitimate research needs.[26]

Second, the public member's presence increases the chance that decisions will be consistent with local community attitudes and values. The decentralized IRB system was established, in part, to allow local ethics to guide research evaluations.[27] In this system, though government regulations set general ethics standards, the standards are interpreted by individual IRBs. Situating ethics review in the setting where research is conducted means that ethical judgments will be sensitive to actual conditions in the community.[28] And members of the general public are well-suited to express the local community "conscience" in deliberating about a study's ethical acceptability.[29] These individuals are also likely to be aware of particular religious, cultural, or economic factors that could affect local reactions to specific research projects.[30] When the potential for harm or rights violations is unusually high, such as in emergency research conducted without prior consent or research in economically disadvantaged areas, it is vitally important to consult people "on the ground" about potential community objections.[31]

Third, the public member can help apply specific ethical and regulatory standards. Public members delineate the real-world meanings of basic ethical concepts, such as respect for persons, beneficence, and justice. For instance, public members are highly qualified to evaluate whether a proposed consent form and process will give individuals the information they need to decide about study participation.[32] Public members help IRBs weed out scientific jargon and impenetrably technical descriptions that appear in informational materials. Public members also add moral and practical insights to the committee's balancing of research risks and benefits. In particular, they may be less likely than scientists and other professionals to assume that advances in knowledge outweigh potential harms to participants.[33] Public members point out when services such as child care are needed to remove barriers to study participation, or conversely, when services or other incentives make study participation too inviting to disadvantaged populations.

The public member's fourth contribution is to promote openness and trust. The research establishment reassures the community by revealing the inner workings of biomedical science to ordinary members of the public.[34] The knowledge that studies will be scrutinized by someone like them reduces community members' suspicions about hidden research improprieties. Besides elevating public confidence in the research endeavor, the public member's participation enhances faith in the government's research oversight system.[35]

The public member's fifth contribution is to foster communication between scientists and the broader community.[36] Public members are translators able to bridge the gap between the worlds of science and ordinary life.[37] When they press investigators and researchers on the committee to describe study goals, procedures, and risks in plain language, public members remind scientists of their responsibilities to communicate with the ordinary people whose study participation and financial support make research possible. Interaction with public members prepares researchers and institutions to respond to media and community inquiries about studies that attract public attention.[38] Public members also help people in the community understand why certain procedures, such as randomization, may be essential in the search for health care improvements.[39]

The public member's sixth contribution is representation. Many writers assign to the unaffiliated IRB member a special responsibility to represent research participants. Thus, they are instructed "to see through the eyes of the patient and imagine what he or she is being asked to go through."[40] Yet public members also receive different messages about their representation responsibilities. Writers describe public members as representatives of potential research "consumers," the general public, the "reasonable ordinary person," poor people and other vulnerable groups, and, most expansively, "patient–subjects, future patients, and the research profession all at once."[41] Moreover, certain patient advocacy and ethics advisory groups believe representatives for specific patient populations, such as people with HIV/AIDS[42] or severe mental illness,[43] should serve as public members on IRBs.

Ambiguous policy directives, together with inconsistent assertions in the literature, create confusion about the public member's role. A responsibility to represent "the general community" is so vague as to be meaningless. The general community includes prospective research participants, patients who stand to benefit from research, research professionals, and a variety of other groups with different interests in the research enterprise. A public member's activities on the IRB could vary substantially depending on which group is represented.[44]

Mixed Motives for Public Oversight

Two general motives appear to underlie policies that endorse public participation in research ethics review. One motive is to improve the ethics of research by adding to the deliberations the values and perspectives of ordinary people. The second motive is to improve public relations by reducing the secrecy and isolation that traditionally characterize research activities.

The historical record reveals that these dual motives have existed since the beginning of the U.S. oversight system. In 1964, an NIH committee recommended that a group of scientists be appointed to draft "a statement of principles relating to the moral and ethical aspects of clinical investigations." But James Shannon, the NIH director at the time, disagreed. Shannon wrote,

> [w]e are inclined to think a broader approach may be necessary. To win general acceptance within not only the medical community but also our society at large, the final statement of principles should probably emerge from a group which includes representatives of the whole ethical, moral and legal interests of society.[45]

Shannon may have hoped that assembling such a mixed group would ensure that the resultant research principles would be consistent with community moral standards. At the same time, Shannon's concern with "winning" general community acceptance may have reflected his desire to protect the research establishment and assure that scientists would be free to continue their work. Thus, including public members in research ethics review "might forestall the possibility of a hostile public reaction against biomedical research."[46] Reassuring the public that research ethics decisions are made not by an insular group of experts, but by a group that includes ordinary people, can also inspire confidence in the review process and the decisions it produces. Consistent with the aim of seeking popular support, public affairs professionals have been enlisted to fill some public member slots on national and state ethics advisory groups.[47]

Commentary accompanying more recent policy requirements for community consultation reveals similar mixed motives. For example, federal officials cited both ethical and public relations justifications for requirements to notify communities of plans to conduct emergency research without consent. Because of the requirements, investigators would "inform individuals within the community about the clinical investigation and permit them to raise concerns and objections."[48] The resulting discussion would alert investigators to potential religious, cultural, and class issues that could create ethical problems with such research.

At the same time, the community consultation rules were issued with public relations in mind. Officials said the requirements were intended "to provide community confidence in the role of the IRB and in its decisionmaking capability. . . ."[49] Indeed, observers report that some research sponsors and institutions have adopted an advertising and public relations approach to implementing the rule, an approach that emphasizes "selling" the study to the community rather than inviting community opinions and adjusting studies accordingly.[50]

Public trust in science and the ethics review system is fine as long as it has a substantive foundation. Similarly, scientific and institutional efforts to garner positive publicity are reasonable if they are backed by meaningful action. The question is whether public participation in its present guise engenders well-founded confidence or unwarranted complacence. How much has the public relations element influenced the structure and operation of research ethics decision making? Do public participants give research ethics review legitimate credibility, or are they mere window-dressing for a system in which the research establishment actually calls the shots?

Limited Authority for Public Participants

Besides exhibiting mixed motives for public involvement in research review, policy officials seem unsure about just how much control "community morality" should exert over the research process.[51] The policies indicate that research should be sensitive to community values, but it is not clear how sensitive. The policies' lack of clarity on this matter, together with rules governing oversight committee composition, suggest that officials are reluctant to give the general community much actual authority to decide research ethics questions.

Like the mixed motives for including public members in ethics oversight, ambivalence about the proper weight of community standards existed at the IRB system's beginnings. In the mid-1970s, philosopher Robert Veatch observed that two different themes predominated in early discussions of research oversight. One theme was that an interdisciplinary group of experts should evaluate the ethics of proposed studies and block research practices that deviated from accepted professional behavior. Those sounding this theme emphasized that reviewers should possess sufficient scientific and clinical expertise to understand the nature and magnitude of research risks, alternative research approaches, and similar technical matters.

The second theme was quite different. Here the emphasis was on an oversight system that included reviewers with what Veatch called "representative or jury skills." Veatch believed that to evaluate a proposal's acceptability to the general community, reviewers had to adopt the perspective of the "reasonable person." Veatch claimed that training and socialization compromise the professional's ability to adopt the reasonable person standpoint in research ethics review. In a point of special interest to ethicists, Veatch argued that even professionals and academics in nonscientific fields are ill-equipped to supply the jury perspective. Veatch characterized professionals as a special class committed to the belief that advances in knowledge are valuable. In contrast, he wrote, people outside the professional realm tend to be less certain that knowledge gains justify risks to research participants.[52]

Veatch doubted that a mixed committee of professionals and public members could truly evaluate a proposal's acceptability to the community. He predicted that even if public members constituted as much as half the group, the committee's ethical judgments would be biased in favor of professional values. In this situation, he thought, determinations would end up midway between what a group of reasonable people would decide and what a professional group would decide. As a result, the mixed committee would be more likely than a group of laypersons to believe that increased knowledge justified risks to research participants. Veatch concluded that only a committee composed entirely of lay members could decide research ethics issues from the vantage point of a reasonable person in the community.[53]

If Veatch was correct, policy decisions to keep public members a minority in the ethics review process allow professional values to dominate. His arguments also lend weight to the suspicion that public participation is designed more to promote public relations than to incorporate public values. We shall see that these misgivings have persisted in the years since Veatch and Shannon first contemplated the community's role in research ethics deliberations.

The Gap Between Aspiration and Reality

More than two decades have elapsed since the IRB system was put into place. During this time, the system has been subjected to extensive scrutiny. Students of the system often conclude that the independent voice of the public participant is rarely heard.

Critics cite three general reasons for public participants' relative silence. In their view, public participants are ineffective because they 1) lack the technical knowledge and independent perspective that would enable them to participate fully in research ethics deliberations, 2) operate in a system that minimizes their power and impact, and 3) lack a definite constituency to guide their contributions to research ethics deliberations.

Critics of existing arrangements for public oversight are unanimous in claiming that the public member does little to disrupt "business as usual" in the research enterprise. For example, a 1998 government report declared, "[f]ew IRBs seem to seek or be able, on a constant basis, to recruit and maintain lay and/or nonaffiliated members who play an active, effective role in helping the IRBs stay focused on their mission of protecting subjects."[54] That same year, a noted authority on clinical research ethics told Congress that public members "often do not become significant contributors to IRB deliberations until they have served for a long enough period of time to develop a relevant ethical and scientific knowledge base. At that point, they generally bring the same concerns and perspectives to the table as their other colleagues on the board."[55] An attorney, summing up his years on an IRB, commented that certain "IRB members were silent or absent—for example the community representative."[56] A layperson serving on a research ethics committee in Australia (which has a system similar to that of the United States) confided, "[t]he main problem in the meetings is thinking how to say what I want to say and make it sound important. Really, the best way is to say what you feel, but it often appears unimportant compared to the other issues."[57]

Empirical data indicate that these perceptions are not unusual. In the mid-1970s, researchers who interviewed IRB members at 61 institutions found that nonscientists "felt generally less active on review committees and perceived themselves to be less influential than other members."[58] In questionnaires and surveys administered a decade later, some public IRB members reported that their performance had been inadequate and others that "although *they* were able to make a contribution and that *their* views were heard and respected, the potential for a less-than-equal role for the unaffiliated nonscientist member certainly was present in the IRB."[59] Members of 86 Australian ethics committees surveyed in the late 1980s reported that public members played a lesser role than others reviewing study proposals. They also rated public members' attendance at meetings as less important than other members' attendance.[60] In another survey of 118 Australian committee members, public members were "rated as significantly less active and less important in their contribution to committee meetings."[61]

Why might public members be functionally absent from the deliberations? One explanation is that they are foreigners to the research enterprise. Newly appointed public members are "strangers in a strange land" faced with a novel language and culture. Initially they may feel lost and barely able to follow the discussion, much less to join it.[62] Through formal or informal training, public members may, over time, develop the expertise necessary to participate in deliberations. But their teachers are usually scientists and clinicians on the committee, who pass on their professional perspectives and values as well. Some writers suggest that to reduce the knowledge gap, committees should fill their public member positions with scientists or clinicians not employed by the institution.[63] Yet many such individuals share the same perspectives and values as researchers on committees. Once again, this strategy puts the public member's purported independent viewpoint in jeopardy.

Critics also attribute the public member's subdued tone to a second source—committee composition and appointment procedures. According to critics, these features of the IRB system operate to minimize the public member's influence. As long as public members constitute a committee minority, they will have little opportunity to counter scientists' values and perspectives.[64] One or two public members will inevitably be unable to offset the scientific and institutional biases that favor research interests.[65]

Besides the lack of influence that comes from their minority status, public members face constraints arising from the appointment process. Public members serve at the invitation of officials at the research institution. In the usual case, IRB chairs and other committee members rely on friends and other informal contacts to suggest possible candidates.[66] Even if an institution adopts more formal appointment procedures, the ultimate choice falls to institutional officials, who are predisposed to choose individuals friendly to the research enterprise. The upshot is that members of the public inclined to question and challenge research practices are unlikely to be appointed.[67]

The third source of public members' relative inactivity is the absence of a definite constituency to guide their participation. Neither the vague policy directives nor the commentaries on IRB oversight clarify the public member's role. Formal policy assigns to the entire IRB a mission to protect research participants. Yet applying the actual policy standards requires committee members to balance participants' interests against the interests served by permitting research to go forward.[68] Scientists and other institutional employees on the committee are predisposed to assign significant weight to the interests of the researchers and future patients who may benefit when studies are allowed to proceed. The unanswered question is whether public members ought to offset this predisposition by giving special consideration to the interests of research participants.[69]

Commentators who lament the absence of a strong public voice on IRBs see this role confusion as a major problem. These commentators claim that role confusion keeps public members from making a distinct contribution and materially compromises their ability to counter institutional self-interest and professional bias in committee decision making.

In sum, critics believe the IRB system does little to encourage authentic public participation in research ethics review. They contend that the existing oversight system puts chief authority for ethics decision making in the research establishment's hands, permits research to proceed with minimal interference, and leaves out ordinary citizens' views of what is ethically acceptable.[70]

Although others reject this critical portrait of research oversight, it has sufficient support to be taken seriously. The data and critical commentary suggest that an independent public perspective is missing from at least some ethics review committees and that the omission might leave research participants worse off than they would be if public members played a more active role. Even though the research oversight system has been reasonably effective in preventing serious incidents of participant mistreatment in recent decades, several inquiries during this period have uncovered ethics violations that IRBs failed to detect or correct.[71] Committees with a significant public presence might have been more successful in ensuring that study participants were adequately informed and that risks to participants were minimized and ethically justified.

Reformers dissatisfied with public members' passivity propose a number of remedies, such as increasing the proportion of public members on oversight committees[72] and improving training opportunities for public members.[73] In the remainder of this chapter, I examine a different potential remedy—adding patient advocates to ethics review. Could more advocacy participation improve the research oversight system? Could advocates supply the technical knowledge, assertiveness, and direction essential to an independent public voice? Or are advocates too narrowly focused and biased in favor of research to add the missing element to ethics review?

Advocates in Research Ethics Deliberations

To date, patient advocacy groups have devoted relatively little attention to research ethics oversight. Most of their energy has gone into promoting research through activities such as fund-raising and lobbying for increased access to clinical trials. Although a few notable exceptions exist,[74] advocates have, for the most part, stayed away from IRBs and debates over whether the rights and interests of research participants are adequately protected.

Why are advocates so scarce in research ethics oversight? In the absence of empirical evidence addressing this question, one can only theorize. My guess is that ethics oversight is comparatively unattractive to advocates because it stresses the negative and disturbing dimensions of biomedical research. Ethics oversight illuminates the dangers of research and the costs of scientific progress. Oversight highlights the unfortunate fact that the search for better treatments requires some people to face unknown risks and receive ineffective interventions. Oversight also reveals the slow and incremental nature of medical progress. Detailed reviews of specific proposals bring home the reality that absolute cures are rare and that advances usually come in the form of small improvements enjoyed by only a limited percentage of patients.

Advocates may find ethics oversight unappealing for other reasons. The IRB review process consumes time and money; thus, it can delay the treatment improvements so desired by advocates. Advocates whose constituents are impatient for cures will seldom want to be identified with a process that can impede scientific work. Ethics oversight does offer advocates an opportunity to serve the subset of their constituents who participate in research. Yet this constituent group is smaller and less visible than the wider group that may benefit from fund-raising and other common advocacy activities. Last, ethics oversight usually addresses research on a broad range of health problems. As a result, advocates may see oversight as less relevant than activities that allow them to focus on specific constituent groups.

Despite all this, good reasons exist for advocates to join research ethics oversight. In my view, both ethics oversight and patient advocacy could benefit from greater exchange. Advocates have much to offer oversight, and oversight has something to offer advocates as well.

Benefits of a Greater Advocacy Role

Patient advocates could be savvy and spirited contributors to research oversight. In previous chapters, we have seen that many activists are proficient in the science and medicine relevant to their advocacy work. These "lay experts" successfully combine technical and personal knowledge to represent constituents' interests in the fund-raising and policy arenas. Their expertise would be a welcome addition to research ethics oversight for at least four reasons.

First, advocates familiar with clinical research issues would be better equipped than most public members to evaluate investigators' proposed disclosure methods, data collection procedures, and other matters affecting study participants. They would be more aware of alternative study methods that would impose fewer burdens on participants. They would be better prepared to cope with the new material that inevitably emerges when specific research proposals are reviewed and discussed.

Second, advocates could bring valuable personal knowledge to research oversight. Because of their close connections to patients, advocates are more likely than are other committee members to appreciate the psychological, familial, and economic conditions that affect research participants. Although most advocates have not worked with the full array of patient groups, many of their specific constituents' concerns apply to people with other health problems as well. In short, advocates are qualified to furnish the personal perspectives professionals are likely to overlook. This is a perspective that can rarely be supplied by the attorneys, ethicists, chaplains, and other nonscientists serving on ethics review panels.

Third, advocates could bring passion, commitment, and energy to ethics deliberations. In contrast to many public members, advocates are likely to be active participants in committee discussions. Advocates are more accustomed to negotiating with clinicians and researchers than is the typical public member. This experience makes advocates less likely to be intimidated by professionals participating in ethics review. Many advocates would not be afraid to question or disagree with elements of a proposed study. Their willingness to speak out would enliven committee discussions and expand the options considered in ethics review.

Fourth, advocates have a ready-made constituency to consult about specific ethical issues. Most advocates have pre-existing relationships with patients, including past and current research participants. Advocates could arrange to talk regularly with patients about research ethics issues. In-depth discussions with people about their research experiences—what participants and their families appreciated and disliked about the process—would give advocates valuable information to contribute to research ethics deliberations. To get a broad picture of the research experience, advocates involved in ethics oversight could ask other advocates for help in reaching study participants outside their ordinary constituencies. These arrangements would give advocates a much closer connection with actual research participants than the typical public member could establish. Advocates skilled in communicating with both expert and lay audiences would also be highly qualified to express participants' concerns in ethics oversight activities.

Besides adding a public perspective to research review committees, advocates could strengthen the public voice in other kinds of ethics oversight. Policy initiatives designed to integrate public perspectives into research ethics decision making tend to follow one of two models. The first model is to include public members on research ethics review or advisory committees. More recent policy initiatives adopt a second model, which requires researchers and review committees to communicate directly with communities that could be affected by specific studies. The U.S. provisions on emergency research without consent and recommendations for community consultation in genetic research follow the second model.

Because policies that adopt the second model for public ethics oversight are relatively new, it is too early to assess their performance. Although many see this model as well suited to elicit the ordinary community's ethical judgments, much will depend on the effort and care devoted to consultation. One major concern is that economic and practical constraints will limit IRBs and investigators to superficial efforts at dialogue.[75] Another concern is that researchers and IRBs will consult too few individuals to obtain a true picture of the community's attitudes and values.[76]

Patient advocates could significantly raise the quality of community ethics consultation. Their distinct knowledge and skills would be just as valuable in community consultation as in research proposal review. Even more useful would be their established relationships with people in the community. Advocates from various patient organizations could cooperate in arranging public discussions of proposed emergency, genetic, and other controversial research projects. Advocates participating in public discussions could ensure that investigators portray studies in a balanced way, without exaggerating benefits or downplaying risks. Advocates could play the translator role in public discussions as well, enhancing communication between researchers and community members.

In sum, the public voice could be stronger if more patient advocates participated in research ethics oversight. At the same time, advocates themselves could benefit from such participation. As IRB members, advocates would spend hours poring over research proposals. This immersion in proposal review would give advocates a deeper understanding of the research process and could be an effective antidote to unrealistic expectations about what research can deliver. The experience could sensitize advocates to the problems of patients outside their ordinary constituencies, which could have a beneficial impact in other advocacy work. Knowledge gained through participating in ethics oversight would help advocates furnish accurate scientific information to constituents and promote improved public understanding of the research process. Increased research knowledge would enable advocates to give constituents more detailed facts about the experience of study participation and supply more meaningful advice to constituents considering study enrollment.

Reservations About Advocates in Oversight

I do not want to suggest that advocacy presents a perfect solution to the public participation problem. The proposal to involve advocates offers neither a panacea nor a guarantee of improvement. Advocacy could fall short for three reasons. First, advocates who participated in ethics oversight would be subject to the same role confusion as other public members. Without clear guidance from policy officials, advocates would share with other public members uncertainty about whether they have a distinct responsibility to represent research participants in ethics deliberations. This uncertainty could diminish advocates' contributions to research oversight.

Second, advocates who joined research ethics deliberations might prefer to represent their specific constituencies. But in many ethics activities, the single-interest approach would be too narrow. As I mentioned earlier, some advocacy groups and policy advisers want IRBs to appoint members to represent particular patient groups, such as people with HIV/AIDS or serious mental disorders. This approach might be suitable for committees in institutions where investigators concentrate their research on specific health problems, but it would be impractical for the majority of IRBs. Most human studies are overseen by institutions whose investigators conduct research on a wide variety of health problems. The "one-disease-one-vote" rule would be too cumbersome for IRBs at these institutions. Adopting such a rule would make committees so large that genuine discussion would be impossible.[77] The rule could also lead to inequities, because powerful and vocal advocacy organizations would probably be more successful in placing advocates on oversight committees.

At the same time, single-interest advocacy would be more suited to the second model for ethics oversight. Community consultation could accommodate a number of advocates representing different patient groups.[78] IRBs could recruit advocates on a case-by-case basis to consult the community about proposed studies affecting specific patient or demographic populations.

Advocates' overall enthusiasm for the research endeavor presents the third and most significant drawback to combining advocacy and research oversight. Previous chapters described advocates' tendencies to convey excessive optimism about scientific progress and the therapeutic benefits of investigational interventions. Many advocates are also preoccupied with securing cures and improved treatments for constituents. If advocates brought these attitudes to ethics oversight, serious problem would arise. Advocates with these attitudes would supply neither a distinct and independent voice nor a check on professional and institutional biases. They would hesitate to demand participant protections that could hinder the research process. They would fail to enhance the committee's knowledge of or sensitivity to participants' situations. They would promote a false sense of security in the community, and, in the worst-case scenario, provide ethical cover for questionable research practices.[79]

Yet these dire prospects are far from inevitable. Many advocates have a sophisticated understanding of research. They would be unlikely to exhibit blind loyalty to the research establishment. Furthermore, through ongoing communications with current and former study participants, advocates could avoid developing a pro-research bias. Such discussions would help advocates achieve a balanced view of research, instead of an overly positive one that would diminish their ability to furnish an independent public perspective.

Next Steps

Not all patient advocates would be suited to oversight work, yet their performance in other areas suggests that many could do an excellent job. Enlisting more advocates for ethics oversight would also be relatively easy to do. This proposal thus has the advantage of being simpler to implement than other suggestions for ethics oversight reform.[80] It would require no formal policy revisions; instead, all that would be needed would be cooperation among advocacy organizations, review committees, and oversight officials.

By attending to two practical matters, advocates and officials could both hasten and elevate the quality of advocacy participation. First, participation in ethics oversight would require a substantial time and energy commitment from advocates. Competing demands and limited budgets could discourage many advocates from shouldering this additional responsibility. To address this problem, officials should consider offering advocates financial support for oversight work. Although compensation could, in theory, reduce an advocate's willingness to challenge researcher and institutional preferences, committed advocates would be unlikely to respond in this way. Indeed, providing compensation would allow advocates to devote more time to fulfilling their oversight responsibilities.[81]

Second, a better system for selecting public participants is needed. Advocates and officials should share authority to appoint public participants. Advocacy organizations could be asked to nominate knowledgeable and assertive individuals for participation in IRB and other oversight activities. Institutional and government officials could then choose participants from among the nominees. The process could include term limits for advocates so that different individuals and patient groups could reap the benefits of the oversight experience, and oversight groups could be exposed to different advocacy perspectives.

Patient advocates had little to do with the policy mandates for public participation in research ethics oversight. Yet their initial absence ought not deter them from joining the process. Oversight presents a rich but neglected opportunity for advocates to serve their constituents and other patients as well. Furthermore, by adding oversight to their repertoire, advocates could give substance to the policy rhetoric on public participation. With their knowledge, passion, and dedication, advocates could fortify the fragile public presence in research ethics deliberations.

7

ADVOCACY FOR
ACCURACY IN
RESEARCH
REPORTING

Whenever a new finding is announced, scientists and clinicians are doing nothing more than making their best guess at the moment. We have to stay tuned, because with more studies we can make an even better guess. Unfortunately, people often infer (and the news media often give the impression) that these guesses and hypotheses are the "truth."[1]

[S]cientific meetings . . . are now becoming more like exercises in public relations organized for the benefit of the media. These meetings, which used to allow the free flow of information between scientists . . . are now typically orchestrated to highlight reports that will clearly appeal to the public or to Wall Street.[2]

The question, of course, is "how to report responsibly," and it is not a question for the media alone.[3]

Access to authoritative information can make the difference between superficial and meaningful advocacy work. Although insights into the personal side of illness stand as advocacy's distinct contribution, advocates also need to know about the technical dimensions of constituents' health problems. To be taken seriously, advocates must have a basic understanding of science and medicine.

Like many nonscientists, advocates gain much of their information from the mass media. Novices to advocacy rely on newspapers, magazines, and the broadcast media for guidance on scientific and clinical developments that affect constituents. Advocates may move on to other information sources, but their constituents continue to depend heavily on the popular media for news about research and treatment innovations.[4]

Thus, advocates have strong reasons to support high-quality reporting about biomedical research. Accurate and realistic accounts of research developments empower advocates in science and policy deliberations. Good reporting helps constituents make informed decisions about health care, research participation, and other dimensions of their personal lives.

Unfortunately, popular reporting on biomedical research leaves much to be desired. For the sake of drama, news stories overstate the clinical implications of study results. Findings from research involving cell cultures and laboratory animals become harbingers of imminent human cures. Complex data susceptible to differing interpretations become the basis for simplistic and misleading health advice.[5] Mass media reporting "alert[s] the public without educating them,"[6] stresses research successes and neglects the disappointments, and pays disproportionate attention to high-profile diseases such as cancer and HIV/AIDS.[7]

Not all popular reporting exhibits serious flaws, yet widespread agreement exists that improvements are needed. Too often, popular media reports foster confusion and misunderstanding among patients and at-risk populations. Too often, journalists and scientists succumb to temptations to exaggerate research outcomes.

Patient advocates are in a good position to challenge these practices. Advocates represent people with the most to lose from irresponsible reporting. As such, advocates are well-situated to demand truthful and realistic research news. They have both the knowledge and the authority to confront journalists and scientists with the real-life consequences of exaggerated research claims. Besides challenging professionals to do better, advocates can counter the negative impact of irresponsible reporting by applying rigorous standards to their own research commentary and guiding constituents to trustworthy research information.

Reporters and Scientists in the Spotlight: Two Illustrations

In May 1998, a *New York Times* article about two compounds called angiostatin and endostatin drew widespread attention. The story began this way: "[w]ithin a year, if all goes well, the first cancer patient will be injected with two new drugs that can eradicate any type of cancer, with no obvious side effects and no drug resistance—in mice."[8] Although the report included numerous caveats and qualifications, its front-page placement and enthusiastic tone suggested that this was a genuine breakthrough in cancer treatment. Many print and broadcast media accounts followed, not all of which contained the cautions in the original report.

The story provoked heated controversy; many claimed it overstated the medical significance of the animal results. Critics called the presentation "unjustly hyped"[9] and "science journalism gone awry."[10] They said the story's compelling lead far overshadowed the reservations that came later.[11] They also complained that the story was based on data reported months earlier in scientific and popular publications.[12] Most disturbing was the way cancer patients responded to the article. Researchers and physicians described being overwhelmed by requests for the "new treatment."[13] They also said some patients were refusing available therapies in favor of waiting for the new agents.[14] Meanwhile, share prices for EntreMed, the biotechnology company developing endostatin, rose from $12 to $83 after the story was published.[15]

This incident serves as a stark reminder of the impact popular reporting can have. Follow-up stories in the *Times* and elsewhere eventually corrected erroneous beliefs about the state of angiostatin and endostatin research. In the meantime, however, some cancer patients and their loved ones were devastated to learn that their hopes of a significant clinical advance were unfounded. Their physicians had the unpleasant task of explaining the preliminary state of the study findings. And in its 1998 Breakthrough of the Year issue, *Science* gave its "award for the most overhyped cancer cure" to "angiostatin and endostatin, whose seemingly magical ability to shrink tumors— in mice—was lauded in *The New York Times* before the treatments were even tested in people."[16]

A year earlier, a different cancer story made the headlines. This one was about a public health recommendation on cancer screening. In this case, disagreement among researchers and clinicians garnered extensive media coverage, with politicians and advocacy groups taking sides and issuing their own pronouncements on the state of the science.

The dispute was over the value of mammography screening to women in their forties. In January 1997, the National Institutes of Health (NIH) convened a consensus development conference to review existing scientific data on the topic. While solid evidence existed that the test saved lives in women aged 50 years and older, the data regarding women from 40 to 49 years old were complex and ambiguous. Mammography detected tumors in women in this age group, but it was unclear whether early detection materially affected death rates. Additional reservations were based on the test's higher error rate for women in their 40s. In this group, mammography has a relatively high rate of false positive results, which trigger unnecessary anxiety, biopsies, and surgery.[17] At the time of the consensus conference, the American Cancer Society and the American College of Radiology recommended routine screening for women aged 40 to 49, but not all medical organizations agreed.[18]

After reviewing the studies and hearing from numerous experts in the field, the panel announced that existing data "do not warrant a universal recommendation for mammography for all women in their forties."[19] Instead, the panel said individuals should decide for themselves whether the possible but uncertain survival benefit from early detection outweighs the possible harm produced by a false positive result.

When the meeting ended, the panel held a news conference to present its recommendation. The immediate response was hostile. Everyone from the director of the National Cancer Institute (a unit of the NIH) to members of the U.S. Senate questioned the panel's conclusions.[20] A radiologist in the audience called the panel report "tantamount to a death sentence for thousands of women."[21] That evening, a major network newscast suggested the panel owed American women an apology for its report.[22]

Over the next few months, the health policy dispute received intense public exposure. Some commentators said opposition to the recommendation reflected mammography's status as "big business in the United States."[23] Others said resistance to the test was motivated more by a desire to save health care costs than by concern for women's health.[24] Advocacy groups expressed different positions on the recommendation, with some defending it as an accurate reflection of the data[25] and others criticizing the panel's failure to issue a more straightforward directive.[26] Still others blamed physicians, health care institutions, and organizations such as the American Cancer Society for "pounding home the message" that mammograms would save younger women's lives without strong evidence that this was so.[27] Meanwhile, the research findings underlying the dispute were "largely garbled in the media."[28]

Journalists, scientists, physicians, advocates, and the public all played a role in this controversy. At the initial news conference, panelists apparently failed to explain and justify the recommendation in terms that could be easily understood by reporters and other nonscientists. With a few exceptions, media reports highlighted the emotional and economic aspects of the dispute without clarifying the state of the science.[29] Certain physicians and professional organizations relied more on emotion than fact to attack a recommendation that threatened their financial interests in maintaining widespread use of mammography.[30] Senators and other nonscientists labeled the report factually erroneous or otherwise unacceptable without an objective basis for their charges.[31] The public reaction reflected women's extreme—and in some eyes, disproportionate—fear of breast cancer, which actually has a low incidence rate in women aged 40 to 50 years.[32] The public outcry also appeared to stem from a wish for simple instructions and easy answers to disease prevention, despite what the best available data show.[33]

These are just two of the many cases in which patients and the public failed to receive an accurate and balanced account of biomedical research findings. What explains this phenomenon? Why do problems persist in the face of widespread complaints and attempts at reform? The answers lie in the pressures on journalists and biomedical professionals to exaggerate research implications. Each group operates in an environment that rewards the over-exuberant reporting about research that can mislead the public.

Pressures to Exaggerate Research Implications

Problems in research reporting rarely involve clear falsehoods. Instead, what is typically at issue are more subtle dimensions of a news story, such as its selection as a newsworthy event, its prominence in a publication or broadcast, the enthusiasm of a headline or introduction, the balance of positive and negative predictions about a new intervention, the number of qualifications included, and the use of certain metaphors and analogies—most familiar are references to "winning" wars and races against disease. Journalists exercise the greatest control over these variables, but the research community has influence as well.

Journalism's Contributions

Although journalists and scientists share certain core ideals, most notably fidelity to the truth, members of the two professions function in very different systems.[34] Deliberation, precision, and specialization are hallmarks of modern scientific practice. But in journalism, speed and versatility are vital. Reporters have a few hours, at most a few days, to prepare stories about complex scientific developments. They do not always have time for the in-depth interviews, fact-checking, and investigative work that yield high-quality research stories.[35] Space or time limits may force them to omit details and nuances that would convey the true meaning of a research advance.[36] What frequently emerge are "sound bite" stories that leave out the qualifiers and contextual features crucial to accurate reporting about research.[37]

Journalists must also be adaptable and flexible in the topics they cover.

General assignment reporters write about multiple subjects. Even those assigned to cover only science or health must write about a wide range of issues and areas.[38] Furthermore, reporters with scientific training and expertise are in the minority. Many journalists lack the background that would enable them to put research in its broader context. Their lack of technical background leaves them insufficiently informed about important concepts, such as peer review, probability, risk, and the incremental nature of scientific progress.[39] It also decreases their ability to question researchers' and sponsors' claims about the value of study findings.[40] Finally, it relegates them to reporting on findings the research community says are significant, rather than what a more independent evaluation would deem newsworthy.[41]

Competition is another factor that affects research reporting. Competition gives journalists incentives to sensationalize research results. Journalists in the same news organization compete with one another to achieve front-page placement or top billing for their stories.[42] News organizations compete with one another to attract the general audience. And because media figures tend to see science as inherently dull, they assume that attracting an audience requires jazzed-up stories.[43]

To "hook" the ordinary person, journalists frequently adopt a human interest perspective on research.[44] News stories may put more emphasis on a patient's or family's response to a study than on an objective assessment of its significance. Another common tactic is to force every research story into a "new hope or no hope" pigeonhole.[45] Use of extravagant language is a third favorite device. Perhaps the clearest example is the almost promiscuous use of the term *breakthrough*. This label has been so broadly and inappropriately applied that some science journalists claim never to use it,[46] and others refer to it as "the b-word."[47] Of course, because the popular media rarely follow-up on the earlier announcements, readers, listeners, and viewers are kept in the dark about all the so-called breakthroughs that fail to pan out.[48]

Extravagant statements also pervade reports about studies suggesting possible associations between disease and a certain lifestyle or genetic characteristic. Such stories seek to attract an audience by dramatizing the dangers and failing to compare them to more familiar health or everyday risks.[49] At times, the quest to enliven such stories is taken to ridiculous extremes, as when a finding that women with submissive personalities had a slightly lower-than-average risk of heart attack was relayed as scientific advice for women to obey their husbands![50]

Reporters are not solely responsible for these defects. Headline writers are especially prone to exaggeration and oversimplification.[51] And editors and producers have perhaps the greatest influence on how research is reported. Few in this group have the scientific training that would enable them to make informed judgments about the quality of science coverage,[52] yet they are the ones who decide what to print, where to print it, and what subjects to cover. Science reporters complain that measured phrases and cautionary statements lead editors and producers to question a story's newsworthiness.[53] What succeeds, instead, are the tried-and-true miracle cure or health panic themes. Reporters also accuse their editors and producers of underestimating the public's interest in and ability to understand less graphic stories about scientific advances.[54]

Finally, economic and personal interests lie at the heart of many of these problems. When journalists adopt the sensationalism that attracts large audiences, profits go up for the companies that employ them. On the other hand, down-to-earth science reporting is not as financially rewarding. Articles on science and health are believed to appeal to readers, listeners, and viewers, but not advertisers. This lack of advertiser interest decreases the economic incentives for news organizations to create special science sections and employ the specialized staff who generally do a better job on research reporting.[55]

Individual reporters may let financial interests affect their work as well. In the angiostatin/endostatin case, for example, questions arose about whether the prospect of a lucrative book contract had influenced the reporter to overstate the agents' potential. (The reporter subsequently withdrew the book proposal.[56]) Temptations to overstate research implications also originate in the "personal insecurity or excessive ambition" of certain reporters "who may overcompensate for normal concerns about protecting one's job security and advancing one's career."[57] These economic and personal interests create incentives for science journalists to go to the edge of, or even overstep, "the boundaries of truth."[58]

Science's Contributions

Biomedical researchers and the institutions that employ them are under increased pressure to publicize study results. Largely because of the patient advocacy movement, biomedical research has a higher public profile than ever before. Patients and the general public pay close attention to announcements from the laboratory. As a result, favorable news reports can boost the image of science and increase public willingness to devote tax dollars to research.[59] Favorable reports can also aid researchers' efforts to obtain more financial support for their work. Government and private sponsors like to see results from their investments, and their general perceptions of past studies can influence future funding decisions.[60] Positive publicity about study results generates good will, donations, patients, and research participants for academic health centers as well.[61]

Though publicity-seeking behavior by researchers is not new, the potential benefits of such conduct are greater than ever before. Revisions in law and policy enable scientists to reap lucrative financial rewards for their discoveries.[62] Moreover, the universities, medical schools, and hospitals that employ them ordinarily share in these rewards. Besides a percentage of the profits produced through commercializing researchers' discoveries, institutions receive a portion of the grants and contract fees awarded to high-profile researchers.[63] Financial stakes are high for the business sector as well. By 1995, 52 percent of the total amount spent for health-related research and development in the United States came from industry sources.[64] This included substantial funding to academic scientists and their employers for biomedical studies.

This increasing commercialization of biomedical research exacerbates the search for publicity, at times producing "blatant attempts to manipulate the media."[65] Industry sponsors, academic and medical institutions, and individual scientists "use the techniques of the business world—press conferences, press releases, video mailings, and Wall Street briefings—to gain or maintain market share or to increase the chances of receiving funding for research."[66] In these contexts, researchers and sponsors may exaggerate claims about study results.[67] Researchers and manufacturer representatives may discuss results without disclosing their industry ties.[68]

Scientific journals also use media coverage to further their financial interests. Many journals depend heavily on corporate advertising for revenues. Some generate vast sums from drug and other product advertisements. According to Lawrence Altman, a well-respected medical reporter, "journals have increasingly become cash cows for the medical societies and companies that own them, with annual profits in the tens of millions of dollars."[69] This situation creates concern that the journals' desires to promote themselves and their advertisers will color their editorial decisions and media interactions.[70]

Scientific journals orchestrate popular media coverage in three major ways. First, they issue press releases that designate certain studies as newsworthy. Releases describe studies in concise, accessible language and spare reporters the time and trouble of finding interesting research on their own. Releases apparently furnish journals with a degree of control over what becomes science news, for a 1998 study found that journal articles described in press releases were more frequently reported.[71] Moreover, releases help keep journals in the spotlight as sources for groundbreaking research.

Two other practices, ostensibly adopted to improve the quality of science reporting, also serve to advance the journals' economic interests. One is the embargo system. Scientific journals that adopt the embargo system release study articles to reporters a week or so before the journals are published. In exchange for this early access, reporters agree not to publish their own stories until just before or at the same time as the journal comes out. Reporters gain added time to decipher and obtain expert commentary on the new studies.

At the same time, the arrangement increases the likelihood that research will be reported as breaking news. As a result, "journals get free publicity, reconfirming them as important because their content is newsworthy."[72]

Journals enforce the embargo by threatening to withhold material from reporters who publish their stories prematurely and by applying a second rule to researchers. To keep scientists from talking to reporters before their journal articles are published, editors refuse to publish studies first reported in the mass media.[73] A few exceptions exist to this rule. Prior to publication, researchers may present data at scientific meetings. If investigators believe their data have urgent public health implications, and journal editors agree, data may be released early. In other circumstances, however, journals will reject any "papers on work that has already been reported in large part."[74]

Journal editors say this secrecy is justified because it allows research to be peer-reviewed for quality before being widely released. The ban on early news stories prevents physicians from "practic[ing] medicine on the basis of newspaper or television reports," allowing them instead to review the scientific publication before deciding whether to adjust their clinical approach.[75] Yet the two rules also preserve the journals' status as cutting-edge science sources, thus maintaining their appeal to readers and advertisers. Although they appreciate having the extra time to digest information and prepare stories, reporters suspect the high-minded public interest justifications mask the journals' true motivations to preserve their prominence and financial well-being.[76]

Difficulties in bridging the gap between science and ordinary life give rise to a separate set of problems that affect research reporting. Scientists are not always skilled or experienced in public communication. They may be unable to explain complex findings or to put them in a broader context for the lay audience. They may be ill-prepared to discourage reporters from adding a sensational twist to study results. They may fail to recognize differences in how scientists and laypersons interpret terms such as "breakthrough" and "negative study."[77]

These shortcomings are a legacy of scientific norms and traditions. Although scientists say they recognize the importance of communicating with the public about research, they are not trained to do so. Moreover, scientists tend to view interactions with the media as distractions from their "real" work in the laboratory. Assisting a reporter engaged in fact-checking or providing expert commentary on a new study takes time away from research. Scientists also fear that in cooperating with journalists, they risk being misquoted or taken out of context, which can lead to professional embarrassment. Furthermore, researchers know that many of their colleagues operate according to an "unwritten code of disdain" for science popularizers.[78] When scientists are reluctant to respond to media inquiries, they make it harder for reporters to determine when study authors or sponsors are making dubious or inflated claims about the significance of their findings.

Last, but not least, many scientists have a strong personal commitment to helping patients. This commitment is understandable and laudable, but it can lead scientists to be more enthusiastic about research findings than is warranted. When "faced with cameras and microphones," such scientists "are overwhelmed by the temptation to make their results live up to the excitement of the moment."[79] The same commitment can color the discussions physicians have with patients about research in the news. A tendency to be overoptimistic with patients can carry over to discussions about the advisability of enrolling in clinical trials or trying unproven interventions recently in the headlines.

In sum, multiple explanations exist for journalists' tendencies to distort and sensationalize health research findings. Similarly, a variety of forces combine to encourage individual researchers, scientific institutions, and scientific journals to dramatize the significance of research results. Unfortunately, when journalists and scientists collaborate to produce misleading research news, "patients are the ones who stand to suffer the most."[80]

The Primacy of Truthtelling

Although they all have incentives to present biomedical research results in a dramatic light, journalists, scientists, and physicians also have professional responsibilities to meet standards of truthful disclosure. Journalists are granted certain privileges and freedoms because we rely on them to keep us aware of important developments that affect our world. In exchange for these privileges and freedoms, journalists are expected to convey news in a context that allows a reasonably informed audience to comprehend the actual significance of an event.[81]

Truthful disclosure is also a fundamental moral principle for scientists. Within the scientific community, of course, researchers rely heavily on one another to report data accurately. But the duty of accurate disclosure extends to the public as well. Public trust in and support for science rest on the expectation that researchers will be unbiased in presenting their results.[82] This expectation covers not only their communications with other scientists but also their statements to reporters. The latter interactions assume particular significance because much of the public receives its information about research from the popular media.

The duty to communicate research results accurately and in context covers physicians as well. Physicians are inextricably linked to the research enterprise as clinical researchers and advisers to patients and journalists seeking information about breaking research news. When physicians meet privately with a patient who has heard about a recent study or discuss a study with a reporter, they deliver information that could influence medical decisions. People cannot make autonomous choices without an accurate picture of how the risks and possible benefits of standard therapies compare with those of novel interventions reported in the news. They cannot make autonomous choices about medical screening, diet, exercise, and other health behaviors without accurate information about the potential harms and benefits of different options. They cannot make autonomous choices without accurate information on the limits of and uncertainties in existing scientific evidence.

The moral principle of respect for persons underlies professional responsibilities to communicate truthfully about research. Their professional expertise and activities give journalists, scientists, and physicians access to knowledge unavailable to the general public. When professionals manipulate information about a study to advance their economic or career interests, to promote the image of science, or even to give hope to patients and families, they show disrespect for the individuals who receive that information. Professionals who distort study information deny members of the general public the opportunity to exercise self-determination in making personal health decisions[83] and in forming opinions about broader public health issues.[84]

Standards for truthful disclosure also rest on the judgment that accuracy will produce the best overall results. Exaggerated optimism about the clinical implications of study findings can have severe consequences to patients and families. Patients who lack a realistic understanding of their prognoses are more likely to undergo burdensome interventions that have little or no chance of extending or improving the quality of their lives.[85] News stories that overstate the implications of research findings reinforce the desperate search for a miracle cure after standard therapies have failed.[86] Such stories give way to dashed hopes once patients obtain more realistic information from their physicians and later more cautious media reports.

The potential negative consequences of inaccurate reporting extend to other health decisions. Mass media messages influence public demand for general health services. News stories can stimulate interest in questionably effective interventions or, conversely, discourage interest in services of demonstrable worth.[87] As the recent explosion in consumer advertising demonstrates, the pharmaceutical industry is convinced that research claims can bolster demand for new drugs. Inflated claims in news stories can have the same impact. Distorted media coverage can also encourage patients and the general public to favor research policies and funding allocations not supported by objective data.[88] Such coverage can blur the distinctions between research and established therapy, thus promoting the therapeutic misconception at both the individual and collective levels.[89]

Finally, journalists, scientists, and physicians who portray research in an overly dramatic light arguably act against their own long-term interests by furthering an erosion of public trust in their institutions. When the genuine significance of an inflated result is revealed, the ensuing disappointment and confusion can fuel a loss of confidence in both the media and biomedical research. Likewise, when people learn that a health recommendation was based more on economic interests than on well-founded data, they lose faith in the research and medical communities and wonder why the media failed to expose the problem earlier.[90] In the long run, such stories can foster cynicism about science reporting,[91] damage the image of science and the media, and diminish enthusiasm for public funding of research.[92]

Advocates As Reform Catalysts

The debate over media coverage is predominately a debate among professionals. Problems with coverage are generally framed as problems for journalists, scientists, and physicians to rectify. Readers, listeners, and viewers are generally regarded as passive information recipients, dependent on professionals to determine how research is presented. Consistent with this perspective, journalists and researchers emphasize the need to devise "more effective ways of getting messages across to an essentially ignorant laity,"[93] and scientists assert that proper reporting on research will "bring people's opinions in line with what scientists think."[94] When the public is mentioned, it is usually with reference to high rates of science illiteracy and the need for improved science education.[95] For the most part, ordinary people are portrayed as subjects of, rather than participants in, research communication.

Patient advocacy organizations have a chance to disrupt this dynamic. Advocates exercise power in other research domains, and they can do so here as well. Rather than waiting for professionals to address deficiencies in research reporting, advocates can both insist on and help determine the needed changes. Besides bringing journalists and scientists face-to-face with the concrete repercussions of inaccurate research reporting, advocates can give professionals a better sense of what constituents are looking for in research news stories. Advocates can also minimize the impact of misleading media reports by guiding constituents and the public to alternative sources of high-quality information about research.

Toward Altered Incentives and Two-Way Communication

Journalists report that complaints from patients and families make a big impression. One editor observed,

[i]f a story promises a cure for a certain disease, readers who have an affected relative and who are desperate for any hope will phone the journalist directly. . . . Having to talk one to one with someone who has a painfully personal interest in a story can be a salutary experience.[96]

Advocates can take advantage of this leverage to change professional behavior. They can urge constituents to call and write letters to news organizations when media stories overstate the clinical implications of research findings. They can write opinion pieces for newspapers and magazines recounting the human costs of excessive claims about research. Coordinated and systematic feedback from advocates and constituents would send a strong message to professionals who violate standards of responsible communication. Regular and vocal public criticism could both deter irresponsible claims and encourage constituents to be more skeptical of popular media accounts.

An organized campaign by advocacy groups would carry even more weight. A campaign joined by thousands of patients and families with different health concerns would be a force to reckon with, one that journalists and the research community would find difficult to ignore. If large numbers of patients and their representatives came together to protest overstated research claims, the temptations to overstate would diminish. If news organizations were confronted with obvious audience dissatisfaction, they would start to see misleading stories as threats to advertising and circulation revenues. Widespread objection to sensationalism would convince editors and producers that the public sees caveats and qualifications as essential to research stories. Negative public reaction would also lessen the appeal of hyperbole and melodrama to reporters intent on career advancement.

Concerted action by advocacy groups would affect the research community as well. If researchers making premature or extravagant claims had to face extensive public skepticism and criticism, the incentives to make such claims would decrease. If overstatement attracted negative rather than positive publicity, individuals and institutions would cease to see it as an effective strategy to build public support for research. If journal editors and public affairs officers knew press releases would receive close scrutiny from knowledgeable and cautious patient advocates, they would hesitate to inflate a study's significance. If claims by corporate research sponsors were monitored by a critical and informed advocacy audience, overstatement would become a less effective business strategy. At the same time, open praise from advocates and constituents for accurate and informative research news would reinforce exemplary professional conduct.

Before launching such a campaign, however, advocates and constituents must develop their own position on what features are desirable and, conversely, unacceptable in news stories. They can begin the process by reviewing what professionals say about these matters. For example, in reacting to the angiostatin/endostatin story, journalist Michael Shapiro wrote:

> Whether a "breakthrough" will herald "the cure" is an inevitable journalistic question. But it is the wrong question—wrong in that it seeks an answer that no responsible oncologist can offer, and wrong in that, by inviting overstatement, it profoundly undermines the great value of the discovery at hand.[97]

Shapiro wants stories on cancer research to emphasize that the disease comes in many forms and requires different treatment approaches. He wants reporters to remind audiences of the probability that a variety of approaches will be needed to produce significant treatment advances, and that, almost always, improvements emerge incrementally over a period of years, sometimes decades. In short, he wants the media to present a new study not as a breakthrough, but as "what it is: . . . one of the thousands of small steps that scientists are taking, along with 'millions of missteps,' that lead to the saving of lives."[98]

Journalists and scientists recommend similar guidelines for stories about research on any serious disorder. When single studies are reported, journalists should put findings into the broader research context and remind people that one study is unlikely to have much effect on patients' clinical options.[99] It is always a good idea to steer clear of breathless, overused phrases such as "scientific breakthrough" and "medical miracle."[100] And stories about research trends can be more informative and less misleading than stories that treat single studies as breaking news.[101]

Other advice applies to reporting on studies that address health risks associated with certain behaviors or genetic characteristics. Journalists should avoid language that suggests that behaviors or genes "cause" disease.[102] To avoid overdramatizing risk estimates, journalists should cite statistics on absolute as well as relative risk. (For example, a new study suggests the disease risk is four times as high as was previously believed, but this is only an increase from one in a million to four in a million people.[103]) For the same reason, they should compare risk estimates to everyday risks, such as driving.[104] When they report on research evaluating the effectiveness of screening tests, such as mammography, they should discuss the test's ability to detect disease *and* extend life and also any risks it imposes, such as unnecessary surgery in the case of a false positive result.[105]

Finally, some guidelines apply to reporting on all types of studies. Reporters should point out when study findings have not yet been peer-reviewed or are limited to a certain sex or age group.[106] They should identify financial or other conflicts of interest that could affect how scientists or sponsors interpret data.[107] They should review graphics and headlines linked to their stories.[108]

To elicit a balanced response to new study findings, reporters should seek comments from a number of experts with different perspectives on the research.[109]

Professional groups believe scientists can do a great deal to improve research reporting as well. In scientific meetings and press conferences, researchers should stress the limits of their findings, describe what additional research will be necessary to clarify clinical implications, and acknowledge important questions a study leaves unanswered.[110] When announcing an agent's effectiveness in animal and other preliminary laboratory tests, researchers should point out that such findings signal only a small possibility that the agent will be safe and effective in humans.[111] In discussions with reporters, scientists should explicitly identify commercial sponsors and disclose any financial interests they have in the research.[112]

Scientists should also pay more attention to their interactions with journalists and the public. They should review news releases and prepare for press conferences and interviews by working with nonscientists to devise accurate and comprehensible study explanations.[113] Researchers should help journalists find qualified expert commentators and accessible ways to present study findings.[114] To avoid misunderstandings, scientists should ask reporters to relay their impression of what has been discussed and read back any statements that might be used as quotations.[115] If a misleading account is published, researchers should request a correction[116] or write a letter to the editor.[117]

Overwhelming agreement exists that journalists should be more knowledgeable about science and researchers more skilled at communication. Professional groups say science seminars ought to be routinely attended not just by reporters, but by headline writers[118] and "media gatekeepers," such as editors, publishers, and news directors.[119] Some professionals want public communication to become an integral part of research, with plain language descriptions accompanying journal submissions and funding agencies supporting researchers for time spent conveying study results to the public.[120]

These ideas and proposals can serve as a starting point for advocates and constituents to develop criteria for good reporting. At the same time, bringing the voices of patients into the debate could lead to new ideas for improved reporting. Advocacy organizations could promote a "bottom up" approach to devising standards for research reporting, one that begins by considering how ordinary people understand health problems and "the context in which they may interpret or apply research findings."[121] Insights gained through this process might end up contradicting the conventional wisdom on what people want to know, including the belief that audiences are attracted only to news about breakthroughs, cures, and dramatic health dangers.

More broadly, advocates could support systematic study of how ordinary people interpret and react to different styles of research reporting. It would be helpful to know, for example, the impact that various cautionary and qualifying statements have on patients, families, and the general public.[122] Without such information, "we cannot say what kind of news coverage is in the best public interest, and recommendations for changes in the behaviour of journal decision makers, media relations staff, and journalists . . . will be based only on opinion and personal judgment."[123]

When Should Biomedical Research Go Public?

Advocates and constituents who develop standards for responsible reporting should devote special attention to the proper timing of research data release. Early data release speeds scientific progress and at times confers a public health benefit. Yet swift release can also trigger unwarranted public excitement or fear in response to study conclusions that are later revealed to be erroneous. Not surprisingly, journalists tend to oppose delays on data release, while the research community is more receptive to them.[124] Yet the timing of data release is not a question simply for professionals. As a major and deeply invested segment of the audience, patients, families, and their advocates have a stake in the decisions as well.

When professionals discuss problems in reporting biomedical research, they point out that the public shares responsibility for those problems. It is unfair, they say, to blame scientists and the media when people let wishful thinking color the way they interpret research news. Research reporting controversies sometimes arise because a longing for "good news" leads readers, listeners, and viewers to gloss over a story's cautionary remarks and concentrate, instead, on its positive elements. Such controversies also arise because the audience wants unambiguous instructions on what they can do to secure longer and better lives.[125]

Biomedical research results are more likely than other scientific findings to have a personal impact on the public. This is especially true for research on life-threatening and other debilitating diseases, such as cancer, HIV/AIDS, Alzheimer's disease, Parkinson's disease, and serious psychiatric disorders. In light of this special public sensitivity, should scientists withhold information about research relevant to serious disease until there is a clear showing of clinical benefit? Should they conceal incremental research advances to keep patients from jumping to conclusions about health implications? Should complicated findings on cancer and other serious health risks be kept under wraps to shield the public from undue confusion and distress?

After the *New York Times* story on angiostatin and endostatin, a cancer patient "undergoing savage chemotherapy" argued for such restrictions. In a letter to the editor criticizing the story, he wrote, "I think the proper time to disclose such drugs as angiostatin and endostatin is after clinical trials are completed and it is determined that they can be released to the general public."[126] On a similar note, a scientist who favors restricting release of animal and in vitro data on environmental carcinogens contended, "until these data are interpreted and evaluated, until the experimental design and significance are reviewed, and until all currently available data on the incidence of cancer in exposed human populations can be integrated, the rush to the press is simply mindless, if not unethical."[127]

These writers want scientists to be empowered to withhold research findings from reporters to protect the public.[128] But the justification for giving scientists this level of paternalistic control is weak. Imposing such broad limits on public data release would be morally inappropriate and practically unworkable.

Although members of the public, most notably patients and their loved ones, are acutely responsive to hopeful research reports, they are not so vulnerable as to lose their status as autonomous moral agents. It is true that the fear and other emotions surrounding serious disease can make it difficult for people to hear the full story about a new study. Yet these emotions are not sufficiently incapacitating to justify concealing news about basic and other preclinical research. Similarly, their strong concern about health and lack of scientific training can make it difficult for people to recognize the limits of and uncertainties in study results. Yet denying the public up-to-date information about ongoing research would be an offensive and patronizing violation of the respect owed to people capable of making their own health and other personal choices.

Furthermore, attempts to exercise paternalism would inevitably fail in today's environment. To keep up with research developments, reporters read scientific journals and attend scientific meetings. Thus, it would be impossible to keep them from learning about studies whose human health implications remain unclear. Many patient advocates also monitor ongoing research and are sufficiently knowledgeable to realize when study findings have possible clinical relevance. Neither journalists nor advocates are likely to support or cooperate with efforts to suppress public disclosure of new research findings. Indeed, attempts to keep data secret could add to the intrigue, spurring unwarranted expectations that disclosure could have avoided.[129]

Nevertheless, journalists, scientists, and physicians should recognize the public's heightened sensitivity to biomedical research news. Although this sensitivity fails to justify paternalistic controls on public communications, it strengthens existing professional responsibilities to resist competing pressures to present research in an unduly dramatic light. Rather than treating patients and the public as children to be sheltered from basic and early-stage clinical research findings, professionals should redouble their efforts to deliver accurate and realistic research news.

A separate question is whether news reports should be delayed to allow research results to be peer reviewed. Modern biomedical research is so complex and vulnerable to misinterpretation that it is risky to rely solely on study investigators to evaluate the quality and significance of their findings. Scientists see peer review as an essential component of the research process; indeed, many characterize a study as incomplete until it has been scrutinized by other researchers.[130] On this view, it is inappropriate for investigators to publish or otherwise make their results widely available until they have taken into account the questions and criticisms of at least a few professional colleagues.

Ideally, the peer review process casts aside poor-quality studies that produce worthless data and detects the limits and weaknesses of studies that merit publication. When peer review conforms to this model, it can prevent inferior science from influencing personal and policy choices. Advocates and constituents thus have material reasons to support requirements for studies to undergo peer review before they are publicly released.

Peer review cannot guarantee quality, however. Few peer reviewers have access to a research group's notebooks and other raw data. This limits the reviewers' ability to detect inadvertent, negligent, or intentional errors in data reporting.[131] Not every peer reviewer invests the time and effort needed to perform an adequate evaluation, and some let personal bias affect their judgments.[132] Finally, the existence of a huge number of scientific journals means that even flawed research can eventually gain acceptance for publication.[133] For these reasons, it would be unwise for advocates and constituents to assume that studies subjected to peer review are error-free. To the contrary, a cautious approach is warranted in evaluating any published study.

Moreover, as we have seen, peer review can be used as a shield to justify publication delays that advance the commercial interests of scientific journals. Patient interests may be compromised when delays are unnecessarily extended so that journals can capture the news spotlight. Although in most cases publication delays have little impact on research progress or public health, exceptions exist. When study authors believe data have immediate and serious public health implications, journal editors have the final say over whether early release is warranted. But because their journal benefits from being the first to publish a high-profile article, editors face a conflict of interest that could affect their decision. Allowing a group of independent scientists and physicians to make this decision would be a better way to ensure disclosure of the (relatively rare) study with serious public health implications.

At a broader level, drawing a line between appropriate delays for peer review and inappropriate withholding of information requires advocates and constituents to consider the degree of control they want scientific experts to exercise in study release decisions. Is it best to postpone public disclosure until a certain number of experts have scrutinized a study for mistakes and misinterpretations? Or would it be better to make the investigators' initial product available to journalists and others, including patient advocates? A third possibility would be to have studies scrutinized by one or two experts and then made widely available for both peer and public assessment.[134]

It is unclear where patient advocates would come out on these questions. Though some advocates are sufficiently knowledgeable and skeptical to evaluate study quality on their own, few constituents are in this category. Thus, some advocates and constituents might see benefits to earlier access, while others would likely prefer a more conservative approach.

To further complicate the issue, independent developments are speeding up distribution of research results. Many scientific journals are moving to electronic publishing, which makes it easier to publicize studies with high scientific or health significance.[135] Some journals post electronic drafts of study articles ("eprints") and allow authors to take reader feedback into account in preparing the final publication.[136] The Internet has exponentially increased public access to other sources of research information, as well.

These trends present both challenges and opportunities to the advocacy community. On the negative side, they increase constituents' exposure to unfounded and exaggerated claims about research findings. On the positive side, they give advocates the ability to construct an independent system for supplying constituents with sound information about biomedical science.

Bypassing the Popular Media

With the growth of patient advocacy groups and the proliferation of information on and off the Internet, the public is no longer dependent on the mass media for research news. Advocacy organizations routinely inform constituents and the public about research. Organizations produce newsletters, brochures, and other materials describing new research findings.[137] Many also have Web-sites advising visitors about research and supplying links to other information resources.[138] An overwhelming number of additional on-line sources cover health issues.[139] For instance, a 1999 article reported the existence of 60,548 Web pages that addressed breast cancer alone.[140] Many of these sources report on research relevant to the health problems they cover.

This explosion of resources is a mixed blessing, for the quality of information is highly variable.[141] Unless they have help in separating the meritorious from the worthless, people will be unable to benefit from their expanded access to information. The tasks for advocates, then, are to produce and direct constituents to trustworthy research material.

Empirical data suggest that patient advocacy groups are trusted news sources. In a 1997 U.S. survey, 93 percent of respondents said advocacy groups were among the most believable sources of health information; indeed, advocacy groups received the same credibility rating as physicians.[142] This high level of trust gives advocates an enormous opportunity to prevent and quickly remedy misunderstandings linked to misleading media stories. At the same time, the public's faith in advocacy organizations imposes a heavy duty of care on advocates who supply research information to the public.

Like professionals, advocates at times succumb to the temptation to exaggerate what research has to offer. It is not unusual for advocates to suggest that research is on the verge of a cure[143] or that an experimental intervention is effective before it has been rigorously evaluated.[144] Like professionals, advocates should refrain from conveying undue optimism when they discuss research developments. Neither the desire to boost constituents' spirits nor the quest to raise money for research should get in the way of research realities. Whether it comes from professionals or advocates, communicating false hope about research is disrespectful and harmful to constituents. Thus, advocates should demand from one another the same degree of accuracy they demand from journalists and researchers. Moreover, like researchers, advocacy groups should disclose financial and other relationships that could affect their portrayal of research developments.[145]

Beyond exhibiting responsible conduct in their own research communications, advocates can review other print and Internet accounts and point constituents to the superior material. For help with this chore, organizations can call on their most knowledgeable lay advocates and on well-regarded researchers and physicians who specialize in the relevant disease area. Besides recommending particular electronic and print sources, advocates can flag the unreliable ones and warn that, because anyone can make claims on the Internet, particular caution is warranted in using this medium.[146] They can urge constituents to discount scientific claims that omit references to peer reviewed studies, come from for-profit organizations, or accompany product or service advertising.[147] Advocacy organizations can maintain libraries to supply reliable and up-to-date research information[148] and recruit staff and volunteers to perform computer searches for people lacking the equipment or skills to do so on their own.[149]

Advocacy groups that create both robust systems for assessing research quality and easily accessible Websites vastly enhance their ability to combat misleading media reports. Groups with these resources can promptly alert constituents and the general public when news stories exaggerate research findings.[150] They can respond similarly when pharmaceutical companies or researchers make questionable research claims. They can be proactive, as well, by offering commentary to reporters[151] and conducting educational sessions for journalists on the scientific, medical, and policy issues relevant to the group they represent.[152]

In sum, advocates have the ability to build a research communications system that treats audiences with respect and sensitivity. They also have the ability to help constituents discriminate between legitimate information and empty promises about research progress. In the end, the best protection against irresponsible reporting is a healthy dose of skepticism, combined with an awareness that genuine treatment breakthroughs are exceedingly rare.[153]

At some level, everyone—people struggling with serious disease, people caring for or mourning an afflicted loved one, scientists and physicians seeking improved treatments, and journalists recounting their stories—wishes for quick and easy answers from research. Yet "whatever may be our wishes, our inclinations, or the dictates of our passion, they cannot alter the state of facts."[154] Biomedical research has contributed to improved health care and will continue to do so. But the public is ill-served when reporters, researchers, or advocates speak of imminent cures and simple solutions to the multitude of ailments that threaten our lives.

8

RESEARCH ADVOCACY TODAY AND TOMORROW

At the end of the twentieth century, patient advocates were an undeniable presence in biomedical research. Advocates transformed research at all levels. They made individual studies more responsive to research participants and to the patients and communities research was intended to benefit. They helped make experimental innovations more widely available to seriously ill people. They persuaded federal officials to adopt requirements for gender and ethnic diversity in study populations. They convinced Congress to boost funding for biomedical research and had a say in how funds were distributed.

At the same time, advocates stayed away from other research issues. They played only a minor role in ethics oversight, perhaps because of its more somber perspective on scientific progress. They remained on the sidelines in debates over how journalists, investigators, and research sponsors publicize study findings.

Their achievements and absences say something about research advocates. Their acts and omissions reveal the strengths, weaknesses, and unexamined features of research advocacy. Their conduct supplies a basis for evaluating advocacy's contributions and for considering where the movement may have gone astray. It points to potential collaborations—and conflicts—between research advocates and research ethicists. It illuminates an array of ethical issues facing advocates and suggests general principles to guide research advocacy. And it sets the stage for what lies ahead.

Old Themes Revisited

In chapter 1, I said I would analyze research advocacy in light of five themes: advocates' positive slant on research, their patient-centered approach to study design and evaluation, variations in the quality and legitimacy of constituent representation, fairness in research planning and policy making, and the relationship of advocacy to research ethics. These themes can now be discussed with greater precision.

The first theme is advocacy's emphasis on the bright side of biomedical research. This attitude is sharply evident in advocacy efforts to expand patients' access to clinical trials and unproven interventions outside the research context. Following the lead of HIV/AIDS activists, patient advocates work to speed drug development and broaden eligibility criteria for clinical trials. They lobby for programs to remove financial and informational barriers to study participation. They portray clinical trials as avenues for patients to obtain cutting-edge treatment. They promise that future patients will be better off if more people participate in today's studies.

Thanks to research advocacy, patients have more freedom to seek help from promising but unproven interventions. Yet stressing research benefits has potential costs as well. The rhetoric of expanded access may mislead research participants, patients, and the public. It may reinforce patients' inclinations to ignore the risks and uncertainties of study participation. It may increase demand for unproven interventions, making it harder to recruit people for studies to determine whether interventions actually work. It may exacerbate patients' disappointment when experimental measures fall short. It may set the stage for public disillusionment with a research enterprise that fails to deliver benefits in rapid fashion.

Advocacy's upbeat portrayal of research is also apparent in the federal funding arena. Advocates seek to influence funding allocation because they see a direct connection between research and constituent benefits. In the advocacy world, funds for research are equivalent to funds for better treatment.[1] In equating the two, advocates add urgency to their requests for research support. Advocates who adopted this approach persuaded Congress to approve significant increases in government funding for biomedical research. Yet the approach also fosters competition among advocacy groups and an arguably disproportionate federal focus on biomedical research, as compared to health care and other important social programs.

Their preoccupation with the positive side of research may also explain advocates' tendency to avoid ethics oversight activities. It may account for their lack of interest in joining ethics review committees and other groups that scrutinize the risks and uncertainties faced by research participants. And it may be one reason they rarely complain when journalists or researchers put an overly positive spin on the significance of study findings.

A patient-centered focus in planning, conducting, and evaluating research is the second advocacy theme. Advocates know how patients and families experience the burdens of illness. This knowledge informs their beliefs about which research questions ought to be investigated and which research proposals should receive funding. Advocates' personal knowledge corrects for the professional myopia that can take scientists too far from the human health mission of biomedical research. Their knowledge adds a different kind of expertise to merit evaluation and priority setting and can promote research programs that yield more meaningful benefits to society. On a smaller scale, their involvement in study planning and data collection and interpretation improves the quality and efficiency of individual studies.

But advocacy's patient-centered approach unsettles some in the research establishment. Critics challenge the idea that advocates are competent to participate in merit review. They fear advocates will undervalue the basic science studies that are the building blocks for clinical progress. They predict advocates will support poor-quality studies on constituents' conditions, or will judge research according to its political correctness. They worry that community representatives will seek undue control over data interpretation and study publication. In short, advocates threaten scientific tradition and ideology when they join peer review and priority setting groups. While the prospects of a more patient-centered research agenda are exciting, advocates will encounter obstacles in promoting this agenda. They will face hard choices as they balance constituent preferences against the demands of good science.

Their patient-centered approach to research may help explain why advocates rarely participate in ethics oversight. Advocates may see ethics oversight as a distraction from their primary mission of promoting benefits to patients, or even as an impediment to improved medical care. Advocates who do participate in ethics oversight may assign highest priority to constituents' needs for better treatments. And advocacy's patient-centered approach may reinforce journalists' and researchers' tendencies to exaggerate the clinical significance of study findings.

The third theme is the varied quality and legitimacy of research advocacy. Research advocates are a diverse lot. Some are extremely well informed about science and medicine relevant to constituents' health problems. These advocates are capable of negotiating with powerful scientists and officials about research priorities and directions. They are capable of making a definite mark on research planning and merit review. If they chose to get involved, they could become leading figures in ethics oversight and media criticism.

For these advocates, the major challenge is to stay connected to the people they represent. Without this connection, they may take positions and agree to policies inconsistent with constituents' needs and preferences. They may lose credibility with their community and be seen as part of the establishment that controls research.

At the other extreme stand advocates with the barest understanding of the scientific and medical dimensions of constituents' health problems. They know only its personal toll. When they recount compelling stories of the hardships patients and families endure, such advocates may persuade officials to channel more resources to research on a certain disease. Yet they may be ineffective in representing constituents in other research areas.

Without basic fluency in the language of research, advocates are likely to remain on the fringes while traditional authorities determine what research is needed, how to conduct it, and whether results affect medical practice. Advocates whose knowledge is limited to the personal experience of disease may be patronized and ultimately ignored by the research teams that consult them. They may be relegated to silence when research proposals are reviewed for merit and ethical acceptability. They may be enlisted as symbolic public participants in a priority-setting process dominated by scientists. They may be manipulated by researchers seeking to advance their own interests in obtaining generous funding for the areas they study. And they may be powerless to respond when the media mislead constituents about the clinical implications of study findings.

Fairness in research policy and planning is the fourth theme relevant to advocacy. A dizzying array of interests are at stake when research decisions are made. Designating certain advocates to represent the community in study planning, merit review, and ethics oversight influences which group and individual interests are taken into account. Expanding patients' opportunities to try experimental interventions outside research decreases the number willing to participate in clinical trials, which in turn affects the quality of treatment available to future patients. Putting money into research on one disease reduces the amount available to study other health problems. Putting money into biomedical research reduces the funds available to study the environment, provide housing to homeless people, and respond to other important social needs.

Not everyone with a stake in the outcomes is represented when patient advocates enter the research arena. Certain groups, such as people with HIV/AIDS and breast cancer, benefit from having experienced, highly effective, and relatively well financed advocates participating in research decision making. At the other end of the spectrum are people with rare diseases, people suffering the diseases of poverty, and others whose advocates lack the knowledge, skills, or resources to exercise influence in research deliberations.

The asymmetries in research representation make it probable that some groups have an unfair advantage in research lobbying. As advocates gain increased opportunities to mold research practice and policy, the disparities will matter even more. The outcome could be a system that pays less attention to the merits of a position than to the strength and visibility of its supporters. To avoid this outcome, officials must devise procedures that give interest groups fair representation in research decision making. Officials must also prepare publicly accessible explanations for specific funding and policy choices. Mandates to disclose reasons for decisions will make it harder for officials to give unfair advantage to particular patient groups.

The fifth theme is the relationship of advocacy to standard research ethics. Research advocates and research ethicists occupy distinct, yet overlapping, territories. Advocates and ethicists are alike in insisting that the interests of research participants and patients must be taken into account when research practices and policies are established. Both believe it is essential to bring the values and concerns of ordinary people to debates over research ethics and policy. Both challenge traditions that give scientists the dominant role in determining the course of biomedical research.

Yet there is discord as well. Advocacy stresses the benefits attainable through research; conventional ethics puts as much or more emphasis on the harms that can result. Ethicists are likely to see certain advocacy activities as disturbingly promotional, and advocates to see ethicists as paternalistic and overprotective. Advocates and ethicists may take conflicting positions on whether community representatives should be empowered to make decisions on behalf of other group members.[2] In some circumstances, advocates may see ethicists as sellouts to the research establishment; in others, ethicists may think the same of advocates.

These differences may be one reason advocates and ethicists have not had much to do with each other. The two groups have operated, for the most part, on parallel tracks, with a few mergers here and there. Does this separation make sense? I would not have written this book if I thought the answer was yes. In my view, advocates and ethicists could benefit immensely from increased interaction. With cooperation, the groups could more effectively promote their mutual aims. They could assist each other in examining the ethical implications of their work. Arguments over conflicting views would benefit the two groups as well, for each would come away with more reasoned positions and an improved understanding of the differences that persist.

Advocacy and Ethics: The Case for Collaboration

People concerned about research ethics should welcome the emergence of research advocacy. At the foundation of modern research ethics is the belief that research practice and policy ought not be decided by scientists alone. Rather, the values and preferences of the broader community should guide research.

In actuality, however, the community is largely excluded from the world of research ethics. Conventional research ethics principles, such as those articulated in the Belmont Report, come primarily from the work of moral philosophers and other theorists. Scholars and practicing ethicists communicate chiefly with one another to ascertain the best approach to real-life research ethics dilemmas. Like other bioethics areas, research ethics "has become its own kind of technical language, its own form of mystification." And "making something complicated is a way of disempowering people."[3]

Professional ethicists are commonly called upon to represent the general community's interests in deliberations about research issues. But professional ethicists are poorly qualified for this task. They are usually employees of a medical school, university, or other institution that is part of the research enterprise. Their colleagues are scientists and clinicians committed to pursuing their research interests. Few ethicists have personal, or even derivative, knowledge of what patients, their families, and the general public think about various research issues.

Advocates are much more capable of bringing this information to research deliberations. The most effective advocates combine an intimate awareness of illness and caregiving with knowledge of the scientific and medical dimensions of disease. With this mixed expertise, they are highly competent to puzzle out the concrete meaning of the abstract ethical principles that guide biomedical research. Moreover, they are vocal and articulate and have strong ties to people who must live with the consequences of research decisions. At this point in time, advocates are better prepared than anyone to represent the community in research decision making.

The emergence of patient advocacy also makes it possible to explore research ethics from the bottom up. Not enough has been done, for example, to ascertain what participation is like for people enrolled in studies. Not enough has been done to discover what participants value, resent, and would change about the research experience. Advocates have knowledge to fill these gaps and ready access to people with even more information about the participant experience.

Here is just one example of how advocates' personal insights could enrich research ethics. Upon learning the findings of the clinical trials on high-dose chemotherapy and bone marrow transplantation for advanced breast cancer, a woman who had undergone the procedure wrote of feeling like a "sacrificial lamb" in an "extreme" experiment. In reflecting on her anger, she admitted that no one had promised the procedure would work and that she had understood the uncertainties. What upset her was that "[n]ot one of the team involved in my bone-marrow transplant . . . even informed me that it had probably been for naught. I guess they just figured someone else would fax me the news report—if they thought about it at all."[4] She observed that this behavior was consistent with the "institutional arrogance" that cancer patients endure, the same arrogance that underlies regular announcements of "yet another next great cure." What would have helped, she and a friend agreed, what would have been "a nod toward dignity," was "a single expression of sorrow or regret" from one of the people performing the procedure. A sign that the outcome "mattered to them even a fraction as much as it mattered to us—would almost have changed everything," she wrote.

I have not seen this suggestion put forward in the standard ethics literature. It has little to do with what standard research ethics emphasizes—autonomous decision making, minimizing risks, and so forth. Yet an expression of sorrow or regret would be completely in accord with the moral principle of respect for persons. It would be an act acknowledging that research results are not simply numbers, but descriptions of real events in real lives. It would be an act that could remind researchers of the human side of their investigations and perhaps encourage greater sensitivity toward participants at other points in the research process.

This is the sort of insight that advocates could contribute to research ethics. Advocates could help ethicists see research from the point of view of research participants and patients in the community. Advocates could be a conduit for participants and patients to talk back to the research establishment and to the ethicists who have become part of that establishment. Advocates could identify hidden difficulties with research practice and policy as well as inventive responses to long-standing problems. They could provide evidence on whether mechanisms such as community consultation in emergency research are achieving their desired aims and devise imaginative remedies for the problems they discover.

Research ethics could benefit advocacy as well. Advocacy raises a multitude of unrecognized and unresolved ethical issues, and the time is ripe for systematic inquiry into these issues. Advocates are a trusted and powerful force in the research arena. Their choices and actions have a significant impact on constituents and others. To preserve their influence and use it wisely, advocates must confront the moral dimensions of their work. The skills and resources ethicists possess would be useful to advocates engaged in self-scrutiny. Ethicists would bring experience with moral analysis and knowledge of an extensive literature relevant to issues facing advocates.

This book is my effort to begin the conversation between ethicists and advocates. In earlier chapters, I examined specific ethical issues that advocates encounter in different facets of their work. Now I step back from the specifics to offer three general ethical principles to guide research advocacy.

Ethical Principles for Research Advocacy

First, advocates should be accurate and realistic when communicating with others about research. In much of their work, advocates convey tidings of hope to constituents and the public. Implicit in the campaign to expand opportunities to try experimental interventions is the message that such options offer deliverance when standard therapies fall short. Implicit in the drive to increase federal funding is the message that research will allow future patients to escape the burdens borne by patients today. Implicit in much advocacy literature is the message that science will at some point triumph over disease.

The optimism is understandable. It undoubtedly provides solace to patients and families and is effective in fund-raising, as well. The problem is that optimism can create unfounded expectations about research prospects. A straightforward appraisal of biomedical progress over the past 50 years reveals a few sudden and significant advances, many incremental improvements, and numerous advances in knowledge that have not yet produced actual health benefits.[5] Thus, talk of complete cures and imminent rescues is almost always disingenuous.

Advocates have a responsibility to be realistic when they speak and write about research. Conveying inflated optimism about what research can deliver deprives patients and families of the facts they need to make research, health care, and other personal decisions. Such optimism can foster public support for research policies and funding allocations that rest on implausible beliefs and can damage advocates' credibility as well.

Overly optimistic communications about research can also damage the patient care system. Optimistic research predictions are an outgrowth of what Daniel Callahan calls the "research imperative . . . the view that medicine has an almost sacred duty to combat all the known causes of death."[6] When the research imperative is at work, it leaves little room for medicine and society to acknowledge and attend to the people science is unable to rescue. Although efforts are under way to humanize nursing home, chronic, and end-of-life care, many patients are still denied comfort and dignity. To the extent that advocates reinforce the attitude that death is "a contingent, accidental event,"[7] an event that research must make every effort to forestall, they help perpetuate a system that neglects chronically ill and dying patients. Forgoing unrealistic optimism about research is one way for advocates to direct attention to the needs of the many constituents the research imperative overlooks.

I am not suggesting that advocates are the sole purveyors of undue optimism about research. An overwhelmingly hopeful tone pervades what many others—scientists, physicians, politicians, and the mass media—say about research. Yet the scope of the optimism makes it even more essential for advocates to assess research realistically.

Of course, it is not easy to be realistic in this context. Advocates discussing research with people affected by serious illness are in a situation that resembles that of physicians informing patients of a poor prognosis. Until relatively recently, physicians avoided disclosing such information out of fear that the truth would be too difficult for patients. Physicians' own discomfort with and lack of training in breaking bad news also made them reluctant to speak frankly. But many physicians changed their behavior as it became clear that the vast majority of people preferred to know the truth, however painful, about their conditions.[8]

Breaking bad news remains one of the hardest tasks for physicians, and one they do not always do well. Yet over time they have learned about balancing honesty and hope in the clinical setting. Their experience offers guidance on striking the appropriate balance in research advocacy. When advocates express unrealistic optimism about experimental and other questionably effective "rescue" options, they may distract patients and families from other care alternatives. Such an approach can also make it harder for patients and families to express and cope successfully with the inevitable painful emotions triggered by a serious diagnosis.[9] Constituents benefit when advocates are prepared and willing to address the full range of possible illness outcomes. Moreover, hope can be attached to goals other than complete recovery. Advocates can forgo unrealistic optimism about the prospects for cure and at the same time encourage hope through exploring and attending to constituents' needs for comfort and supportive care.[10]

Research advocacy should be guided by a second ethical principle: appreciation for the diversity of constituents. Like advocates, constituents are a heterogeneous group. Some constituents have the necessary self-assurance, education, and economic wherewithal to be savvy research consumers. Others, however, do not. As a result, a "one-size-fits-all" approach to advocacy risks compromising the interests of certain constituents.

Savvy research consumers are the primary beneficiaries of the Food and Drug Administration's expanded access programs, the government-sponsored clinical trials database, improved insurance coverage for clinical trial participants, and other measures that enlarge the menu of alternatives available to people seeking to ameliorate or avoid serious disease.[11] Constituents in this group are sufficiently educated to understand information about the potential harms and benefits of, and alternatives to, research participation. They are equipped to locate and decipher additional information relevant to decisions to enter research or try innovative therapies. They are less likely than others to be misled by claims in the popular media. In short, they are as prepared as anyone can be to "face uncertainty, take responsibility for decisions, and communicate clearly"[12] in the research setting.

At the other end of the continuum are constituents with more limited abilities to benefit from expanded information and access to experimental alternatives. These individuals lack the education and resources to navigate the research world on their own. They are intimidated by the medical system and prone to follow the suggestion of anyone wearing a white coat. They would prefer to have someone else advise, even decide, on the option that would be best for them. People in this group benefit from programs designed to protect patients and research participants from being harmed by experimental interventions. They benefit from safeguards that prevent researchers and others with their own agendas from taking advantage of vulnerable or misinformed individuals. These constituents are served by more paternalistic research practices and policies.

Advocates face difficulties in representing constituents on different parts of the continuum. Programs and policies that advance the interests of some constituents could be detrimental to others. Access programs that serve the astute, experienced patient may draw in others less able to appreciate the trade-offs involved. But restrictions designed to protect patients from undue risks may be condemned as arrogant, disrespectful, and offensive by those who feel equipped to make the decision themselves.

Even language choices can be complicated. As I noted earlier, advocates prefer to substitute the term *research participant* for the traditional *research subject. Participant* connotes an active contributor owed the same respect as scientists and clinicians participating in a study. On the other hand, the term implies that all participants possess equal power and control. In most biomedical studies, however, professionals inevitably have the upper hand. They are the ones who decide what procedures will be performed and the ones most aware of the risks and uncertainties involved. People enrolled in research are truly *subjects* in the sense that they are dependent on researchers for information and protection. Thus, use of the term *participant* is a double-edged sword. It can encourage people to be active and assertive research volunteers. At the same time, it can promote false confidence among participants and undermine investigators' sense of responsibility for the well-being of the individuals they study.[13]

The challenge for advocates is to take into account constituents' various interests and situations. It is fine to promote the liberty of constituents who are prepared to exercise it, but safeguards are also needed for those who lack the means to protect themselves. Advocacy efforts to date seem most tailored to confident, well-educated patients able to take full advantage of their expanded opportunities. Advocates should supplement this approach with programs to assist constituents who are not in this position.

Achieving this goal will require a more fine-grained approach to research advocacy. It will require extensive communication with a wide range of constituents. It will require gathering detailed information on matters such as constituents' abilities to access the Internet and their interest in learning more about experimental options. It will require asking constituents what services would assist them in choosing whether to enroll in a trial or try an unproven intervention outside the research setting. Collecting this information will give advocates an enriched picture of constituents' interests, one that comes from constituents themselves. Advocates armed with this information will be able to promote research practices and policies that benefit a broad range of constituents.

The third ethical principle is to reject parochialism in research advocacy. Advocates guided by this principle will explore the full array of policies and services that could benefit constituents. These advocates will support policies and resource allocations that advance constituents' interests in obtaining established health care as well as promising experimental interventions. These advocates will not concentrate solely on research advocacy if significant numbers of constituents lack access to standard treatments of proven benefit. And in campaigning to secure insurance coverage for patients in clinical trials, these advocates will endorse measures to make both trials and established treatments more accessible to uninsured patients.

Advocates who adopt this principle will recognize that an exclusive focus on generating health benefits through research would harm constituents. Accordingly, in pursuing treatment gains through expanded research programs, they will not overlook the rights and welfare of the study participants who make improved treatment possible. In advocating for increased trial enrollment opportunities, they will support measures that promote informed and voluntary decisions to enroll. They will recognize that low-income and uninsured constituents may participate in studies to gain needed services and will work to rectify the problem.

Advocates who apply this principle will take into account patients with other serious conditions as well. On first glance, such an approach may appear to conflict with advocates' responsibilities to pursue the most advantageous outcomes for their constituents. Yet often no real conflict exists. Constituents themselves are vulnerable to other health problems, and most have family and friends at risk for or affected by a wide range of diseases. Thus, constituents have interests in maintaining research and other programs designed to assist people with a variety of conditions.

As a practical matter, an inclusive approach may also be best for constituents. Single-minded research advocacy is often ineffective. As we saw in chapter 5, competition among advocates lobbying for federal research funds can be detrimental to fund-raising efforts. Moreover, officials are unlikely to respond to advocates who cannot tie their positions to broader public policy goals.[14] As a guide for government lobbyists observed, "viewing the world through [a single-interest] lens causes an astigmatism—a shortsighted prescription for decreasing effectiveness, to the point where one is only heard, not listened to."[15]

Last, single-interest research advocacy raises ethical questions. Groups engaged in analogous activities set limits on zealous partisanship, and research advocates should, too. As noted in chapter 5, the American League of Lobbyists urges both professional and citizen lobbyists to "temper the advocacy role with proper consideration for the general public interest," and to "fairly represent all points of view."[16] Similarly, elected officials considering policies that promote constituents' interests are not free to ignore people outside their districts.[17] And though lawyers are strongly obligated to champion their clients' interests, they may not completely disregard their moral obligations to others.[18]

One rationale for setting limits on partisanship in other settings applies to research advocacy as well. Strong partisanship is unfair when not everyone with an interest in the outcome is adequately represented. Partisanship is permitted in the lobbying context on the assumption that other interest groups are also represented. According to one Senate aide, lobbyists "may have an obligation to ascertain that [their] arguments are made in a format in which the [congressional] staff member has an opportunity to hear the other side."[19] When elected officials consider policies that will affect people both inside and outside their districts, favoring residents' interests is unfair if nonresidents lack representation.[20] The lawyer's duty of zealous representation exists in the framework of an adversarial system that ensures representation for each party. And even in the adversarial system, extreme zealousness on behalf of a client may be morally inappropriate when the opposing side lacks the resources or capacity to mount an equally vigorous case.[21]

The challenge for advocates is to engage in forceful research representation without losing sight of the bigger picture. Advocates and constituents should consider how research lobbying fits into their organization's general mission. They should determine the proper priority to give research funding and policy in light of constituents' overall interests.

At a broader level, advocates should support measures that promote fair representation for all affected groups in research funding and other policy deliberations. Advocates should also consider collaborating to devise a comprehensive plan for meeting the nation's health needs. Such a plan could include a range of projects to benefit diverse constituencies. Organizations could coordinate lobbying activities to promote these projects. A collaborative approach would reduce unseemly and self-defeating competition among interest groups. Moreover, an alliance of advocacy organizations would be a powerful force in shaping government, industry, and charitable support for research, health care, and other social services.

Some advocates will undoubtedly take issue with these three ethical principles and with positions taken elsewhere in this book. Others will label the analysis incomplete because it fails to cover a noteworthy topic or omits material relevant to a topic that is discussed. To these advocates I say, "Speak up!" Your point of view is essential to developing a robust account of research advocacy ethics.

A second advocacy contingent may reject the very idea of an inquiry into research advocacy ethics. Advocates have an overwhelming number of urgent claims on their energy and resources. Why should they add ethics to this nearly endless list? I offer three reasons for doing so.

The first is self-interest. Advocates who ignore the ethical implications of their work risk losing the respect and trust of others. Advocacy activities are monitored by constituents, the media, and the general public. Advocates who fail to identify and think through ethical issues will be ill-prepared to respond when their conduct is questioned or criticized. If this happens too often, they could lose constituent support and influence over research and policy decisions.

Their responsibilities to constituents give advocates a second reason to consider ethics. Advocates are obligated to act in the best interests of the people they serve. Ethical analysis can help advocates meet this obligation. The research ethics literature explores the nature and scope of patients' and research participants' interests and offers guidance on balancing those interests in different research and policy settings. By attending to ethics, advocates can reduce the chance that they will overlook or assign disproportionate value to particular constituent interests.

The movement's success creates a third reason to incorporate ethics into research advocacy. Advocates' actions have major consequences not just for constituents, but for other patients, families, and the general public. This power to affect others gives advocates a responsibility to examine the moral dimensions of their work.

Preparing for Advocacy's Next Phase

In the twenty-first century, advocates will confront a multitude of novel questions and demands. Although not all are foreseeable, it is possible to discern the outlines of a few. Three topics in particular merit attention.

One is whether HIV/AIDS activism should continue as the model for research advocacy. As the first modern disease activists, HIV/AIDS advocates set the tone for those who followed. The success of HIV/AIDS advocacy prompted other disease interest groups to adopt similar goals and strategies. Now it is time for advocates to examine the virtues and pitfalls of the HIV/AIDS advocacy approach.

Several features of HIV/AIDS advocacy remain worthy of imitation. Most prominent is an emphasis on acquiring scientific and medical knowledge. Although full-fledged scientific expertise is unnecessary, advocates do need to develop a basic understanding of research and clinical information relevant to disease. Acquiring such knowledge enables advocates to lobby and negotiate more effectively on behalf of constituents.

The grassroots character of HIV/AIDS advocacy is another feature with persistent appeal. The grassroots approach keeps advocates aware of the personal side of illness. Through encouraging substantial local involvement, advocates stay in touch with constituents' individual concerns. Besides providing compelling stories that draw public attention to their struggles, individual constituents educate advocates, researchers, and officials about the shortcomings of available therapies, symptoms and problems that merit research attention, difficulties encountered in study participation, and other topics relevant to research.

One additional attribute of HIV/AIDS advocacy is worth preserving: the refusal to regard experts as infallible. Traditional patient advocacy organizations exhibited substantial, if not absolute, deference to researchers. HIV/AIDS activists proved that patient advocates could be legitimate and persuasive research critics. They demonstrated that informed patient advocates could actively and positively contribute to the research process. Advocates should strive to continue and expand their work as research collaborators.

Other features of HIV/AIDS activism seem less suited to future research advocacy. The primary research aims of HIV/AIDS activists were increased funding and access to experimental interventions. These aims made sense in the context of an emerging infectious disease that attacked a relatively young and otherwise healthy population. In this context, it was reasonable to expect that an intensified research campaign would yield material clinical benefits in a relatively short time. Sadly, however, most of the other major afflictions that threaten people in developed countries present more formidable and enduring barriers to scientific progress.

Organizations should adapt their research advocacy to the patients they serve. Certain deviations from the HIV/AIDS advocacy model might be in order for organizations that represent people with cancer, heart disease, chronic obstructive lung disease, dementia, and other common serious conditions. As I argued earlier, creating unrealistic expectations for speedy cures can be harmful to constituents and the patient care system. Such an approach can disappoint and embitter constituents and the public when anticipated advances fail to materialize.

HIV/AIDS activism sounds a second cautionary note for future research advocacy. Although several of the activist challenges to the research establishment had merit, others did not. As discussed in chapter 3, certain HIV/AIDS activists had second thoughts about selected aspects of federal policies that liberalized access to unproven agents. In addition, some HIV/AIDS activists eagerly embraced disease theories and interventions that were later discredited.[22] These advocates learned the hard way that assertions and anecdotes cannot substitute for rigorous research and that initially exciting interventions often fail to live up to their promise. These experiences ought not dissuade future research advocates from scrutinizing research conventions, but should stand as a warning to avoid haste and oversimplification in reaching their positions.

HIV/AIDS activism offers a third lesson for the next phase of research advocacy. Most activist leaders were young and middle-aged, relatively affluent and well-educated, white gay men. Not surprisingly, their perspectives influenced their research advocacy. They sought practices and policies that failed to take into account the views and interests of other at-risk groups. When members of the latter groups began their own lobbying efforts, they were not always welcomed by established activists. Indeed, some early HIV/AIDS activists were charged with exhibiting the sort of elitism and authoritarianism they once criticized in the biomedical establishment.[23]

These events highlight the importance of staying alert to constituent diversity. Advocates who fail to consult with a representative sample may end up promoting policies and practices that disadvantage certain constituents. Such advocates also invite criticism from those whose views are left out. When this occurs, advocacy must be put on hold while internal disagreements are addressed. Sometimes dissenters form their own group to challenge and compete with the original organization, which can detract from the general goal of advancing patients' interests. The HIV/AIDS experience demonstrates the value of enlisting a diverse group of constituents to guide advocacy efforts.

Another topic relevant to advocacy's next phase is the changing character of clinical research. Industry sponsorship of clinical research is on the rise. Pharmaceutical and medical device companies are developing a host of new products that require human testing. The demand for research participants has never been higher, and commercial sponsors have come up with new techniques to meet this demand.

In one major change, businesses are hiring free-standing contract research organizations—disparagingly referred to as "research factories"[24]—to manage clinical trials. These organizations enlist community physicians both to recruit their patients for trial participation and to administer the trials. Physicians are reimbursed for the time and expenses associated with data collection. For physicians facing declining revenues as a result of managed care, clinical trials have emerged as a means to offset financial losses.[25]

The changing research climate can be perilous for patients. When their personal physicians bring up the possibility of enrollment, patients may mistakenly assume that study participation will be an extension of ordinary clinical care. Patients may also enroll to avoid irritating someone whose good will they want to maintain.[26] Physicians who rely on research remunerations to supplement their incomes may consciously or unconsciously put pressure on patients to enroll.[27] Some physicians may go so far as to expose medically unsuitable patients to unacceptable risk by enrolling them in studies contrary to formal exclusionary criteria.[28]

These problems are magnified when corporate sponsors offer physicians incentives above and beyond the usual reimbursement fees. If study enrollment is proceeding too slowly, sponsors offer bonuses to physicians who recruit new participants.[29] Sponsors also pay physicians "finder's fees" for recruiting patients to participate in studies conducted elsewhere.[30] In such cases, temptations to encourage enrollment and downplay risks become more difficult to resist.

Coupled with the avid pursuit of study participants is an increasingly overtaxed research oversight system. Institutional review boards (IRBs) must evaluate increasing numbers of study proposals, often without adequate staff or funding.[31] Because proposals receive less individualized attention, ethical problems may go undetected. Resource constraints have always limited IRB monitoring of study procedures, and the increased committee burdens make such monitoring nearly impossible. Academic institutions have become more dependent on commercial sponsors for research support, and some fear this will make IRBs hesitant to question the ethics of industry-sponsored studies.[32]

Concern about the quality of ethics review extends to independent committees acting as IRBs. These freestanding IRBs, though not a new development, are playing a more prominent role in research oversight. They review proposals for companies, hospitals, and universities.[33] Most are for-profit entities supported by payments from their clients. This financial arrangement triggers worries that business interests will compromise the independent IRB's commitment to engage in thorough and rigorous ethics oversight.

The altered research enterprise threatens research integrity as well.[34] Empirical studies suggest that industry-funded trials tend to produce results favorable to a trial sponsor's new drug.[35] Corporate research sponsors may try to suppress[36] or substantially delay[37] publication of findings unfavorable to their products. Data collection and reporting may be manipulated by researchers who have direct financial interests in a study's outcome.[38]

Research quality may also be jeopardized in studies that require community physicians to perform tasks outside their ordinary areas of expertise. Critics of community-based research question whether inexperienced physician–investigators will detect the often subtle effects of study drugs.[39] Products approved for clinical use based on poor-quality data could turn out to be risky or ineffective.

Future research advocacy must adjust to the emerging "market economy for research."[40] The advocacy response should target constituents, government officials, and executives in the private sector. First, advocates should alert constituents to the growing role of financial incentives in the research enterprise. In light of the increasing involvement of community physicians in research, it is vitally important for constituents to understand the differences between receiving clinical care and participating in a study. Advocates should also warn constituents to be on guard for unexpected problems that may arise in the use of newly approved drugs and devices.

Policies addressing the threats posed by increased commercialization also have important implications for constituents. Advocates should support rig-

orous institutional and regulatory conflict of interest rules that minimize investigator bias in conducting, reporting, and reviewing research. They should
insist on adequate government monitoring to assess the safety of research
participants and the accuracy of data reported in industry-sponsored studies.
They should demand a heightened federal commitment to ensure that IRBs
have sufficient resources and authority to carry out their ethics oversight
responsibilities.[41]

To date, advocacy has focused on government research policies and funding
decisions. But with industry controlling a growing percentage of biomedical
research, advocacy belongs in the private sector as well. Indeed, at this point,
research advocacy may be most needed in the private sector. Moreover, as
consumer representatives, advocates have a reasonable chance to succeed in
influencing corporate conduct.[42]

Private sector research advocacy should target several areas. Commercial
sponsors should be notified that deviations from research ethics standards are
unacceptable. Advocates should offer assistance to companies seeking to meet
ethical standards, such as advice on techniques that would promote informed
decision making by trial participants.

Advocates should also address research priority setting in the private sector.
Advocates should press industry sponsors to develop medications and other
innovations that will fill significant gaps in existing therapy. Advocates should
speak out against the pharmaceutical industry's use of resources and study
volunteers to develop drugs substantially similar to agents already on the market.[43] Advocates should urge pharmaceutical and other companies to put corporate good citizenship above profits when compelling health needs are at
stake. In this vein, advocates should encourage businesses to sponsor and
cooperate with government programs that promote research on rare diseases
and the health problems of poor people in the United States and worldwide.[44]

Research advocacy should be directed to nonprofit foundations as well. Although foundations supply a relatively small portion of the total funding for
biomedical research, their contributions rose substantially during the 1990s.
Like government and industry, foundations set priorities for research funding.
Some foundations engage in extensive study before deciding what areas to
support; others are governed largely by donors' personal interests in particular
fields or diseases.[45] Certain foundations that support biomedical research have
endowments of more than several billion dollars and are capable of having a
material impact on research progress. Foundations with such extensive resources arguably assume responsibilities to consider the public good in distributing resources.[46] Advocates should urge foundations to perform systematic
and careful analyses of unmet health needs before allocating funds for biomedical research.

Finally, advocacy organizations face internal issues created by the increased commercialization of biomedical research. It is not unusual for drug companies and other businesses to seek alliances with patient advocacy organizations, and these requests are likely to occur more frequently in the changing research environment. Businesses typically offer an organization payment or a donation in return for the right to use the organization's name in marketing activities.[47] Such an exchange generates financial support for advocacy activities. At the same time, however, it creates a potential conflict of interest for advocacy organizations. Consumers may interpret use of an organization's name as a product endorsement by patient advocates they admire and trust. To avoid the ethical and legal problems associated with such arrangements, advocacy organizations should adopt conflict of interest policies. Such policies should define when disclosure of corporate support is sufficient to address ethical concerns and when support must be rejected as incompatible with the advocacy mission.

Besides their forays into the corporate and nonprofit worlds, future research advocates will enter debates over the appropriate use of novel biomedical technologies. Advocates already have begun to participate in policy discussions on xenotransplantation,[48] stem cell,[49] and gene transfer[50] research. These research areas present examples of intricate and politically charged questions that will confront twenty-first-century research advocates.

Innovations in biomedical research require advocates to develop new kinds of scientific expertise. Advocates who seek to become full participants in policy debates over xenotransplantation, stem cell, and gene transfer research must understand something about the fields of molecular biology, genetics, immunology, and infectious diseases, among others. Acquiring such knowledge is an arduous but necessary step in developing defensible positions on the ethical and policy issues raised by these research innovations.

The goal of xenotransplantation, stem cell, and gene transfer research is to assist seriously ill patients unable to benefit from standard therapies. When the research aim is to rescue desperately ill patients, it is tempting to move quickly to the first human trials.[51] The problem is that researchers may seek to proceed before there are sufficient animal and other preliminary data to suggest that an intervention will be safe and potentially beneficial for humans. As patient representatives, advocates can play an important role in preventing premature attempts to try novel interventions in humans.

Advocates will also be forced to balance patients' interests in pursuing novel interventions with broader societal concerns. Xenotransplantation carries a remote but potentially serious risk of transmitting animal diseases to the human population.[52] Stem cell research could yield advances that dramatically extend the human life span, creating severe resource constraints for future generations.[53] Gene transfer research could make it possible to enhance normal human functioning, but such enhancements are likely to be expensive and available only to the wealthy.[54] Certain forms of stem cell research necessitate destruction of human embryos, and gene transfer research is likely to involve human embryos as well.[55] Thus, advocates contributing to policy formation in these fields will be forced to take positions on the politically controversial subject of human embryo research.

To date, most advocates who have participated in debates on xenotransplantation, stem cell, and gene transfer research have supported continued work in these areas. They have emphasized patients' interests in obtaining therapeutic benefits from these procedures. They have argued that safety considerations fail to warrant moratoria on xenotransplantation[56] and gene transfer research in humans.[57] Most have opposed restrictions on stem cell research to prevent destruction of human embryos.[58] They have also disagreed with proposals to constrain xenotransplantation, stem cell, and gene transfer research to protect broader societal interests.

These positions are likely to be tested in the coming years. Advocates who promote early human testing may draw criticism if innovations later prove dangerous and ineffective.[59] Advocates who support human embryo research may encounter unaccustomed opposition from religious organizations and certain constituents as well.[60] Advocates may find themselves in the midst of contentious debates over the extent to which patients' interests ought to trump broader social concerns.

Of course, not all of advocacy's future challenges will involve the frontiers of biomedical research. Everyday research advocacy will generate plenty of challenges as well. Future advocates may have difficulty sustaining constituent and public enthusiasm if research fails to deliver dramatic treatment improvements. A deeper understanding of research trade-offs and uncertainties may lessen patients' willingness to participate in clinical research, particularly in phase I and other studies that offer little or no chance of direct benefit to participants.[61] Researchers and officials in various settings may regard advocates primarily as public relations tools and turn a cold shoulder to patient-centered reforms. Politicians[62] and entrepreneurs[63] may attempt to manipulate research advocacy to advance their own interests.

Biomedical research both reflects and influences the values of the society in which it occurs. I hope that advocates will persist in their fierce campaign to put patients' interests at the forefront in research deliberations. But I also hope that advocates will strive for a thoughtful, careful approach to constituent representation. I hope they will show compassion to all patients in need and cultivate alliances rather than divisions among advocacy groups. I hope they will recognize that research can be a siren song that diverts attention from our failure to supply proven treatments and living assistance to all patients in need. I hope they will acknowledge the limits of research as a means to advance constituents' interests and speak frankly about these limits to patients and the public.

Practicing advocacy with these considerations in mind will not be easy. Incorporating ethics will complicate the advocacy mission. Yet advocacy is likely to be the better for it. In the end, attention to ethics will build the most enduring foundation for future research advocacy.

NOTES

Chapter 1

1. "Postal Service, American Express Initiatives Benefit Breast Cancer Research," *Journal of the National Cancer Institute* 90 (1998): 1866; Jodi Wilgoren, "Compassion and Hope in 60 Miles of Shared Moments," *New York Times*, 13 June 2000, D10; American Express, "Help Fight Breast Cancer," *New York Times*, 23 September 1999, A12; Lisa Belkin, "Charity Begins at . . . The Marketing Meeting, the Gala Event, the Product Tie-In," *New York Times Magazine*, 22 December 1996, 40–46, 52, 55–56; and Constance Holden, "Record Home Run Benefits Cancer Research," *Science* 283 (1999): 483.

2. Erik Stokstad, "From Junk Bond King to Cancer Crusader," *Science* 283 (1999): 1100–1103. Indeed, advocacy organizations see celebrity representatives as vital to research fund-raising. See Claudia Kalb, "Stars, Money and Media Crusades," *Newsweek*, 22 May 2000, 58–60.

3. Katherine Q. Seelye, "Gore's Plan for Success in '00: An Array of Solid Positions," *New York Times*, 29 July 1999, A16; David Malakoff and Eliot Marshall, "NIH Wins Big As Congress Lumps Together Eight Bills," *Science* 282 (1998): 598–599.

4. Elizabeth Pennisi, "Patients Help Track Down Disease Gene," *Science* 288 (2000): 1565, 1567; Gina Kolata, "Parents Take Charge, Putting Gene Hunt Onto the Fast Track," *New York Times*, 16 July 1996, B5, B7. In a variation on this theme, a cystic fibrosis advocacy group is supplying $30 million to a biotechnology company for work on drug development. See Eliot Marshall, "Disease Group Invests in Do-It-Yourself Drugs," *Science* 288 (2000): 1715, 1717.

5. Tony Hope, "Medical Research Needs Lay Involvement," *Journal of Medical Ethics* 24 (1998): 291–292. For a discussion of developments in the United Kingdom, see Christine Hogg, *Patients, Power & Politics* (Thousand Oaks, California: Sage Publications, 1999).

6. Bruno Latour, "From the World of Science to the World of Research?" *Science* 280 (1998): 208–209.

7. Tessa Tan-Torres Edejer, "North–South Partnerships: The Ethics of Carrying Out Research in Developing Countries," *British Medical Journal* 319 (1999): 438–441.

8. Federation of American Societies for Experimental Biology, "Accelerating the Pace of Discovery at the National Institutes of Health," 29 May 1998. Accessible on the Internet at http://www.faseb.org/opar/Principles.html.

9. Denise Drevdahl, "Coming to Voice: The Power of Emancipatory Community Interventions," *Advances in Nursing Science* 18 (1995): 13–24.

10. Iain Chalmers, "Further Suggestions for Other Terms to Describe Participants Are Needed," *British Medical Journal* 318 (1999): 1141.

11. Abigail Zuger, "Patient Suffers From Connotationitis," *New York Times*, 31 August 1999, D5.

12. Petra Boynton, "People Should Participate In, Not Be Subjects of, Research," *British Medical Journal* 317 (1998): 1521.

13. Belkin, "Charity Begins," p. 46. Although patient activism itself was not a new phenomenon, HIV/AIDs activists were the first to target and successfully alter biomedical research practice and policy. See Steven Epstein, *Impure Science: AIDS, Activism, and the Politics of Knowledge* (Berkeley: University of California Press, 1996), pp. 8–14.

14. C. P. Gross and K. A. Sepkowitz, "The Myth of the Medical Breakthrough: Smallpox, Vaccination, and Jenner Reconsidered," *International Journal of Infectious Disease* 3 (1998): 54–60.

15. Peter J. Cohen, "The Placebo is Not Dead," *IRB: A Review of Human Subjects Research* 20 (March-June 1998): 8.

16. Senator Bill Frist, "Setting Biomedical Research Priorities at the National Institutes of Health," *FASEB Newsletter*, December 1997. Accessible on the Internet at http://www.faseb.org/opar/newsletter/dec97/4×12×97.html.

17. Representative Ernest Istook, "Research Funding on Major Diseases is Not Proportionate to Taxpayers' Needs," *Journal of NIH Research*, (August 1997): 26–28.

18. Paul Appelbaum, et al., "False Hopes and Best Data: Consent to Research and the Therapeutic Misconception," *Hastings Center Report* 17 (April 1987), 20–24.

19. Nancy King, "Experimental Treatment: Oxymoron or Aspiration?" *Hastings Center Report* 25 (July-August 1995), 6–15.

20. Special Advertising Supplement, "Diabetes . . . How Kids Cope, Critical New Research," *New York Times Magazine*, 26 September 1999, 61–80.

21. This is the slogan popularized by the Susan G. Koman Breast Cancer Foundation. Accessible on the Internet at http://www.breastcancerinfo.com.

22. Alexander Capron, "Ethical and Human-Rights Issues in Research on Mental Disorders That May Affect Decision-Making Capacity," *New England Journal of Medicine* 340 (1999): 1432.

23. Institute of Medicine, *A Review of the Department of Defense's Program for Breast Cancer Research* (Washington, DC: National Academy Press, 1997), 63.

24. Nancy Maull, "Science Under Scrutiny," *Harvard Magazine* (March–April 1997): 27.

25. Amy Langer, "The Role of Advocacy in Cancer Research: Not a Monster," *Cancer Investigation* 15 (1997): 500–502.

26. Epstein, *Impure Science*, p. 342.

27. Charlotte Williamson, "The Challenge of Lay Partnership," *British Medical Journal* 319 (1999): 721–722.

28. Office of Public Liaison, "NIH Director's Council of Public Representatives," 2000. Accessible on the Internet at http://www.nih.gov/about/publicliaison/COPR.htm.

29. National Commission for the Protection of Human Subjects of Biomedical and Behavioral Research, *The Belmont Report: Ethical Principles and Guidelines for the Protection of Human Subjects of Research* (Washington, DC: Government Printing Office, 1979).

30. David Rothman, *Strangers at the Bedside* (New York: Basic Books, 1991), pp. 182–189.

31. Rothman, *Strangers at the Bedside*, pp. 30–100.

32. "Federal Policy for the Protection of Human Subjects," *Federal Register* 56 (1991): 28,012–28,018.

33. Baruch Brody, *The Ethics of Biomedical Research: An International Perspective* (New York: Oxford University Press, 1998).

34. Rebecca Dresser, "Time for New Rules on Human Subjects Research?" *Hastings Center Report* 28 (November-December 1998): 23–24.

35. Nancy King, Gail Henderson, and Jane Stein, "Relationships in Research: A New Paradigm," in *Beyond Regulations: Ethics in Human Subjects Research*, ed. Nancy King, Gail Henderson, and Jane Stein (Chapel Hill, North Carolina: University of North Carolina Press, 1999), p. 13.

36. Susan M. Wolf, ed., *Feminism and Bioethics* (New York: Oxford University Press, 1996).

37. Kathryn Montgomery Hunter, *Doctor's Stories: The Narrative Structure of Medical Knowledge* (Princeton: Princeton University Press, 1991).

38. Nancy Kass, et al., "Trust: The Fragile Foundation of Contemporary Biomedical Research," *Hastings Center Report* 26 (September–October 1996), 25–29.

39. Carl E. Schneider, *The Practice of Autonomy* (New York: Oxford University Press, 1998).

40. Leo Alexander, "Medical Science Under Dictatorship," *New England Journal of Medicine* 241 (1949): 39–51. I thank my colleague Stephen Lefrak for referring me to Alexander's comments on advocacy organizations.

41. "Federal Policy for the Protection of Human Subjects," p. 28,015.

42. Food and Drug Administration, "Protection of Human Subjects: Informed Consent," *Federal Register* 61 (1996): 51,538.

43. Council for International Organizations of Medical Sciences, *International Ethical Guidelines for Biomedical Research Involving Human Subjects* (Geneva: CIOMS, 1993), p. 25.

44. Eric Juengst, "Group Identity and Human Diversity: Keeping Biology Straight from Culture," *American Journal of Human Genetics* 63 (1998): 673–677.

45. Amy Gutmann and Dennis Thompson, *Democracy and Disagreement* (Cambridge, Massachusetts: Harvard University Press, 1996), pp. 84–94.

Chapter 2

1. Herbert R. Spiers, "Community Consultation and AIDS Clinical Trials, Part I," *IRB: A Review of Human Subjects Research* 13 (May–June 1991):8.

2. Institute of Medicine, *A Review of the Department of Defense's Program for Breast Cancer Research* (Washington, DC: National Academy Press, 1997), p. 94.

3. Andrea Cornwall, "Towards Participatory Practice: Participatory Rural Appraisal (PRA) and the Participatory Process," in *Participatory Research in Health: Issues and Experiences*, ed. Korrie de Koning and Marion Martin (Atlantic Highlands, New Jersey: Zed Books, 1996), p. 94.

4. Benjamin Freedman, "Equipoise and the Ethics of Clinical Research," *New England Journal of Medicine* 317 (1987): 141–145.

5. Kenneth J. Rothman and Karin B. Michels, "The Continuing Unethical Use of Placebo Controls," *New England Journal of Medicine* 331 (1994): 394–398.

6. Steven Epstein, *Impure Science: AIDS, Activism, and the Politics of Knowledge* (Berkeley: University of California Press, 1996), pp. 253–254.

7. Steven Epstein, "The Construction of Lay Expertise: AIDS Activism and the Forging of Credibility in the Reform of Clinical Trials," *Science, Technology, & Human Values* 20 (1995): 417.

8. The underlying scientific issues concern the acceptable trade-offs between the need to keep extraneous factors from distorting an agent's effects (which creates pressure for narrow eligibility criteria) and the need to produce data that apply to a reasonable percentage of people affected by the condition being studied (which supports including a broader range of affected people). See National Advisory Mental Health Council Clinical Treatment and Services Research Workgroup, *Bridging Science and Service* (1998), pp. 28–31. Accessible on the Internet at http://www.nimh.nih.gov/research/bridge.htm.

9. Epstein, *Impure Science*, p. 339.

10. Karen Stabiner, *To Dance With the Devil: The New War on Breast Cancer* (New York: Dell Publishing, 1997), pp. 61–65. See also Irene M. Rich, et al., "Perspective from the Department of Defense Breast Cancer Research Program," *Breast Disease* 10 (1998): 33–45.

11. Institute of Medicine, *Review of DOD Program*, p. 59.

12. Ibid., pp. 62–63.

13. The Integration Panel has a role similar to that of the institute and center advisory councils at the National Institutes of Health. I describe the advisory council role in chapter 4.

14. Institute of Medicine, *Review of DOD Program*, p. 62.

15. Ibid., p. 63.

16. Ibid., p. 98.

17. National Breast Cancer Coalition Press Release, "Fran Visco Elected to Chair Integration Panel of the Department of Defense Breast Cancer Research Panel," 27 January 1999. Accessible on the Internet at http://www.natlbcc.org/press/dod.asp.

18. National Action Plan on Breast Cancer, "Consumer Involvement," 1999. Accessible on the Internet at http://www.napbc.org.napbc/consumer.htm.

19. National Breast Cancer Coalition, "Project LEAD—Leadership, Education and Advocacy Development," 1999. Accessible on the Internet at http://www.natlbcc.org/LEAD/lead_info_new.asp.

20. National Breast Cancer Coalition, "World Conference on Breast Cancer Advocacy Influencing Change," 1999. Accessible on the Internet at http://www.natlbcc.org/meetings/world/backgrnd.asp.

21. Rajesh Tandon, "The Historical Roots and Contemporary Tendencies in Participatory Research: Implications for Health Care," in *Participatory Research*, ed. de Koning and Martin, pp. 19–26.

22. Andrea Cornwall and Rachel Jewkes, "What Is Participatory Research?" *Social Science and Medicine* (1995) 41: 1667–1676.

23. Ibid., p. 1668.

24. Arthur Chen, et al., " 'Health Is Strength': A Research Collaboration Involving Korean Americans in Alameda County," *American Journal of Preventive Medicine* 13(Suppl. 2) (1997): 93–100.

25. Heather Goodare and Richard Smith, "The Rights of Patients in Research," *British Medical Journal* 310 (1995): 1277–1278.

26. S. Jody Heymann, "Patients in Research: Not Just Subjects, But Partners," *Science* 269 (1995): 797–798.

27. Bruce Agnew, "NIH Invites Activists Into the Inner Sanctum," *Science* 283 (1999): 1999–2001.

28. Robert Cook-Deegan, "Inner Sanctum," *Science* 284 (1999): 589.

29. Tammy O. Tengs, "Planning for Serendipity: A New Strategy to Prosper from Health Research," Progressive Policy Institute Health Priorities Project Policy Report No. 2, July 1998, p. 5.

30. Elizabeth E. Tolley and Margaret E. Bentley, "Training Issues for the Use of Participatory Research Methods in Health," in *Participatory Research*, ed. de Koning and Martin, pp. 50–61.

31. Heymann, "Patients in Research," p. 797.

32. Iain Chalmers, "What Do I Want from Health Research When I Am a Patient?" *British Medical Journal* 310 (1995): 1318.

33. Ibid., p. 1317.

34. Chen, et al., "Health Is Strength," p. 97.

35. Chalmers, "What Do I Want from Health Research," p. 1317.

36. Goodare and Smith, "Rights of Patients," p. 1278.

37. National Advisory Mental Health Council Workgroup, *Bridging Science and Service*, p. 48

38. Ibid.

39. "In Quotes: NIMH's Hyman on Mental Health Research," *Science & Government Report*, 15 August 1998, p. 3. Advocates also argue that medical journals should condition publication on a showing that clinical studies incorporated community consultation and should include consumers among the reviewers who decide whether studies merit publication. Heather Goodare and Sue Lockwood, "Involving Patients in Clinical Research," *British Medical Journal* 319 (1999): 724–725.

40. National Commission for the Protection of Human Subjects of Biomedical and Behavioral Research, *The Belmont Report: Ethical Principles and Guidelines for the Protection of Human Subjects of Research* (Washington, DC: Government Printing Office, 1979).

41. Gary B. Melton, et al., "Community Consultation in Socially Sensitive Research," *American Psychologist* 43 (1988): 576–577.

42. Tri-Council Policy Statement, "Ethical Conduct for Research Involving Humans: Context of an Ethics Framework," 1998. Accessible on the Internet at http://www.mrc.gc.ca/ethics/english/intro03.htm.

43. David M. Chavis, Paul E. Stucky, and Abraham Wandersman, "Returning Basic Research to the Community," *American Psychologist* 38 (1983): 431.

44. Carol P. Herbert, "Community-Based Research as a Tool for Empowerment: The Haida Gwaii Diabetes Project Example," *Canadian Journal of Public Health* 87 (1996): 110.

45. Goodare and Smith, "Rights of Patients," p. 1278.

46. National Cancer Institute, Director's Consumer Liaison Advisory Group, "Meeting Summary," 17 December 1997. Accessible on the Internet at http://deainfo.nci.nih.gov/ADVISORY/dclg/17dec97.htm.

47. Freedman, "Equipoise and Ethics," p. 144.

48. Jason Karlawish and John Lantos, "Community Equipoise and the Architecture of Clinical Research," *Cambridge Quarterly of Healthcare Ethics* 6 (1997): 385–396. This idea also underlies the practice of appointing patient representatives to independent data and safety monitoring committees. These committees evaluate study data as

they are collected to determine whether there is enough information to demonstrate that one intervention is superior. If so, the study may be discontinued early. Such decisions require committee members to balance the potential harms to participants of continuing the study against the potential harms to future patients of an inaccurate evaluation. Patient representatives on committees can supply a community perspective on whether there is sufficient uncertainty about the data to justify continuing the study. Malcolm A. Smith, et al., "Role of Independent Data-Monitoring Committees in Randomized Clinical Trials Sponsored by the National Cancer Institute," *Journal of Clinical Oncology* 15 (1997): 2736–2743.

49. Karlawish and Lantos, "Community Equipoise," pp. 390–391. See also Heather Sutherland, Eric Meslin, and James Till, "What's Missing from Current Clinical Trial Guidelines? A Framework for Integrating Science, Ethics, and the Community Context," *Journal of Clinical Ethics* 5 (1994): 297–303.

50. Martha A. Carey and Mickey W. Smith, "Enhancement of Validity Through Qualitative Approaches," *Evaluation and the Health Professions* 15 (1992): 107–114.

51. Lynn Blanchard, "Community Assessment and Perceptions: Preparation for HIV Vaccine Efficacy Trials," in *Beyond Regulations: Ethics in Human Subjects Research*, ed. Nancy King, Gail Henderson, and Jane Stein (Chapel Hill, North Carolina: University of North Carolina Press, 1999), pp. 85–93.

52. National Commission for the Protection of Human Subjects of Biomedical and Behavioral Research, *Belmont Report*, pp. 5, 7.

53. Dennis Willms, et al., "Participatory Aspects in the Qualitative Research Design of Phase II of the Ethnocultural Communities Facing AIDS Study," *Canadian Journal of Public Health* 87 (1996): S15.

54. Ann Macaulay, et al., "Participatory Research with Native Community of Kahnawake Creates Innovative Code of Research Ethics," *Canadian Journal of Public Health* 89 (1998): 105–108.

55. Epstein, *Impure Science*, pp. 253–264.

56. Ibid., pp. 258–262. See also Rebecca Dresser, "Wanted: Single, White Male for Medical Research," *Hastings Center Report* 22 (January-February 1992): 24–29.

57. Nancy King, Gail Henderson, and Jane Stein, "Regulations and Relationships: Toward a New Synthesis," in *Beyond Regulations*, ed. King, Henderson, and Stein, pp. 213–224. Chapter 6 discusses advocacy participation in IRBs and other research ethics oversight activities.

58. Herbert Spiers, "Community Consultation and AIDS Clinical Trials: Part III," *IRB: A Review of Human Subjects Research* 13 (September-October 1991): 3–7. This attitude has emerged among people who supply tissue for genetic research. As scientists increasingly seek patents and other financial rewards for products developed through such studies, more research participants reportedly want to share in the proceeds. Gina Kolata, "Sharing of Profits Is Debated As the Value of Tissue Rises," *New York Times*, 15 May 2000, A1, A17.

59. Epstein, "Construction of Lay Expertise," p. 426.

60. Philip B. Gorelick, et al., "Establishing a Community Network for Recruitment of African Americans Into a Clinical Trial," *Journal of the National Medical Association* 88 (1996): 703.

61. Janet A. Seeley, Jane F. Kengeya-Kayondo, and Daan W. Mulder, "Community-Based HIV/AIDS Research-Whither Community Participation? Unsolved Problems in a Research Programme in Rural Uganda," *Social Science and Medicine* 34 (1992): 1089–1095.

62. Rachel Nowak, "AIDS Researchers, Activists Fight Crisis in Clinical Trials," *Science* 269 (1995): 1666–1667.

63. Carol Levine, Nancy Neveloff Dubler, and Robert J. Levine, "Building a New Consensus: Ethical Principles and Policies for Clinical Research on HIV/AIDS," *IRB: A Review of Human Subjects Research* 13 (January-February 1991): 8.

64. Agnew, "NIH Invites Activists," p. 2000.

65. Ibid.

66. Mary K. Anglin, "Working from the Inside Out: Implications of Breast Cancer Activism for Biomedical Policies and Practices," *Social Science and Medicine* 44 (1997): 1403–1415.

67. Agnew, "NIH Invites Activists," p. 2000.

68. Herbert, "Community-Based Research," p. 110.

69. Ibid., pp. 110–111.

70. Ibid. See also Blanchard, "Community Assessment and Perceptions," p. 93

71. Alan F. Benjamin, "Contract and Covenant in Curacao: Reciprocal Relationships in Scholarly Research," in *Beyond Regulations*, ed. King, Henderson, and Stein, p. 60.

72. Sue E. Estroff, "The Gaze of Scholars and Subjects: Roles, Relationships, and Obligations in Ethnographic Research," in *Beyond Regulations*, ed. King, Henderson, and Stein, pp. 76, 78.

73. Renee C. Fox, "Contract and Covenant in Ethnographic Research," in *Beyond Regulations*, ed. King, Henderson, and Stein, p. 69.

74. Ronald P. Strauss, "Community Advisory Board-Investigator Relationships," in *Beyond Regulations*, ed. King, Henderson, and Stein, p. 97.

75. Ibid., p. 95. See also Chavis, Stucky, and Wandersman, "Returning Basic Research," p. 29.

76. Chen et al., "Health Is Strength," p. 98.

77. Ibid.

78. Cornwall and Jewkes, "What Is Participatory Research?" p. 1674.

79. Ibid.

80. Shubhada J. Kanani, "Introducing Participatory Research to University and Government Health Systems: Some Experiences from India," in *Participatory Research*, ed. de Koning and Martin, pp. 229–237.

81. D. V. Mavalankar, J. K. Satia and Bharati Sharma, "Experiences and Issues in Institutionalizing Qualitative and Participatory Research Approaches in a Government Health Programme," in *Participatory Research*, ed. de Koning and Martin, pp. 216–228.

82. Epstein, *Impure Science*, p. 13.

83. Epstein, "Construction of Lay Expertise," p. 424.

84. Anglin, "Working from the Inside Out," p. 1411. See also Alessandro Liberati, "Consumer Participation in Research and Health Care," *British Medical Journal* 315 (1997): 499.

85. Envy of the economic benefits people receive for their research work can be another source of hostility in poor communities. See Seeley et al., "Community-Based HIV/AIDS Research," p. 1093.

86. Epstein, *Impure Science*, p. 349. Institute of Medicine, *Review of DOD Program*, p. 100.

87. Sandra R. Oliver, "How Can Health Service Users Contribute to the NHS Research and Development Programme?" *British Medical Journal* 310 (1995): 1318–1320.

88. Cornwall and Jewkes, "What Is Participatory Research?" p. 1673. For discussion of the special difficulties in defining groups for purposes of genetic research, see Eric

Juengst, "Group Identity and Human Diversity: Keeping Biology Straight from Culture," *American Journal of Human Genetics* 63 (1998): 673–677.

89. The Institute of Medicine committee that reviewed the DOD program questioned the rationale for the different definitions and suggested that if a survivor's viewpoint was important in first-level review, it would seem to be equally important in making final funding recommendations. Institute of Medicine, *Review of DOD Program*, p. 94.

90. Cornwall and Jewkes, "What Is Participatory Research?" p. 1673.

91. Ibid.

92. Strauss, "Community Advisory Board-Investigator Relationships," p. 97.

93. Cornwall and Jewkes, "What Is Participatory Research?" p. 1673. See also Bebe Loff, "Violence in Research," *Lancet* 355 (2000): 1806.

94. Korrie de Koning and Marion Martin, "Participatory Research in Health: Setting the Context," in *Participatory Research*, ed. de Koning and Martin, pp. 12–13.

95. Denise Drevdahl, "Coming to Voice: The Power of Emancipatory Community Interventions," *Advances in Nursing Science* 18 (1995): 19.

96. Anglin, "Working from the Inside Out," pp. 1411–1412.

97. Epstein, "Construction of Lay Expertise," p. 420.

98. Vikki A. Entwistle, et al., "Lay Perspectives: Advantages for Health Research," *British Medical Journal* 316 (1998): 464.

99. Epstein, "Construction of Lay Expertise," p. 499.

100. Epstein, *Impure Science*, p. 343. As noted earlier, the DOD Breast Cancer ResearchProgram assigns consumer representatives with scientific training to panels outside their areas of expertise to help representatives maintain their distinct community perspectives.

101. Herbert Spiers, "Community Consultation and AIDS Clinical Trials: Part II," *IRB: A Review of Human Subjects Research* 13 (July-August, 1991): 5.

102. For example, the Breast Cancer Research Foundation's logo states "A Cure in Our Lifetime." Breast Cancer Research Foundation, "Help Fight Breast Cancer," *New York Times*, 23 September 1999, A12.

103. Melton et al., "Community Consultation in Socially Sensitive Research," p. 578.

104. Keith A. Wailoo, "Research Partnerships and People 'At Risk': IV Vaccine Efficacy Trials and African American Communities," in *Beyond Regulations*, ed. King, Henderson, and Stein, p. 106.

105. Oliver, "How Can Health Service Users Contribute?" p. 1319.

106. Philip R. Reilly, "Rethinking Risks to Human Subjects in Genetic Research," *American Journal of Human Genetics* 63 (1998): 682–685.

107. Seeley, Kengeya-Kayondo, and Mulder, "Community-Based HIV/AIDS Research," p. 1095.

108. Entwhistle et al., "Lay Perspectives," p. 465.

109. Ibid., p. 463.

110. In determining whether a study presents an acceptable balance of risks and potential benefits, for example, individuals belonging to the group that will be asked to participate are usually the best community representatives. See Karlawish and Whitehouse, "Is the Placebo Control Obsolete in a World After Donepezil and Vitamin E?" *Archives of Neurology* 55 (1998): 1420–1424.

111. An exception in this area is the DOD Breast Cancer Research Program, which requires first-level consumer reviewers to be nominated by an organization with relevance to breast cancer and chooses reviewers based on the quality of their applications.

112. The National Childbirth Trust, a British organization that represents people

using pregnancy and childbirth services in the National Health Service, provides a model approach. To obtain members' views, advocates discuss research issues in the organization's journal and at membership conferences. They also distribute materials to local groups to elicit community opinions on matters such as priority areas for research about pregnancy and delivery. Oliver, "How Can Health Service Users Contribute?," pp. 1319–1320.

113. Tolley and Bentley, "Training Issues," p. 50.

114. See also Helen Schiff, "Inner Sanctum," *Science* 284 (1999): 590–591, voicing advocates' strong support for innovative approaches to research on breast cancer.

115. Agnew, "NIH Invites Activists," p. 2000.

116. Monitoring and evaluation could suggest modifications to improve the process. For example, consumers might be more effective if they were asked to apply review criteria specifically geared to their abilities and expertise. The National Institute for Mental Health has adopted this approach, instructing consumer panelists to evaluate proposals based on "public health significance and/or innovation; on the feasibility of plans for recruitment, retention, and follow-up of subjects; on outreach efforts to special populations; and on protection of human subjects." National Institute of Mental Health, "Invitation to Individuals to Serve as Public Participant Reviewers on NIMH Scientific Review Groups," 1998. Accessible on the Internet at http://www.nimh.nih.gov/grants/pubpart1.htm.

117. Macaulay et al., "Participatory Research with Native Community," p. 107.

118. Entwhistle et al., "Lay Perspectives," p. 465.

Chapter 3

1. Herbert Spiers, "Community Consultation and AIDS Clinical Trials: Part III," *IRB: A Review of Human Subjects Research* 13 (September-October 1991): 7.

2. Laura Wexler, "Studies of Acute Coronary Syndromes in Women—Lessons for Everyone," *New England Journal of Medicine* 341 (1999): 275.

3. National Institutes of Health, "Clinical Trials Database," 1999. Accessed on the Internet at http://www.nih.gov/health/trials/index.htm. Perhaps in recognition of its promotional tone, officials had removed the shopping reference by the time the database made its formal debut in February 2000. National Institutes of Health, "Clinical-Trials.gov," February 2000. Accessible on the Internet at http://clinicaltrials.gov/.

4. Michael Milken, "Testimony to the Senate Subcommittee on Labor, Health and Human Services and Education Appropriations," 16 June 1999. Accessible on the Internet at http://www.senate.gov/appropriations/labor/testimony/mlkn6_16.htm.

5. Sheila Shulman and Jeffrey Brown, "The Food and Drug Administration's Early Access and Fast-Track Approval Initiatives: How Have They Worked?" *Food and Drug Law Journal* 50 (1995): 503–531.

6. Herbert Spiers, "Community Consultation and AIDS Clinical Trials: Part II," *IRB: A Review of Human Subjects Research* 13 (July-August 1991): 2, 3.

7. Steven Epstein, *Impure Science: AIDS, Activism, and the Politics of Knowledge* (Berkeley: University of California Press, 1996), pp. 222–226.

8. Although the program is popularly referred to as "compassionate use," this is not official FDA terminology. The phrase is misleading in suggesting that allowing seriously ill persons to try unproven measures is a merciful act. As this chapter discusses, such measures can have negative as well as positive effects on patients.

9. Food and Drug Administration, "Investigational New Drug, Antibiotic, and Biological Drug Product Regulations; Treatment Use and Sale," *Federal Register* 52 (1987): 19,466–19,477.

10. Food and Drug Administration, "Expanded Availability of Investigational New Drugs Through a Parallel Track Mechanism for People with AIDS and Other HIV-Related Diseases," *Federal Register* 57 (1992): 13,250–13, 259.

11. Food and Drug Administration, "Investigational New Drug, Antibiotic, and Biological Drug Product Regulations; Procedures for Drugs Intended to Treat Life-Threatening and Seriously Debilitating Illnesses," *Federal Register* 53 (1988): 41,516–41, 524.

12. Food and Drug Administration, "New Drug, Antibiotic, and Biological Drug Product Regulations; Accelerated Approval," *Federal Register* 57 (1992): 58,942–58, 960.

13. Ibid., pp. 13, 234–13, 242.

14. Shulman and Brown, "Food and Drug Administration's Early Access and Fast-Track Approval Initiatives," p. 506.

15. Robert Temple, "Are Surrogate Markers Adequate to Assess Cardiovascular Disease Drugs?" *Journal of the American Medical Association* 282 (1999): 790–795.

16. "Report of the Public Health Task Force on Women's Health Issues," *Public Health Reports* 100 (1985): 73–106.

17. Nancy Kass, "Gender and Research," in *Beyond Consent: Seeking Justice in Research,* ed. Jeffrey Kahn, Anna Mastroianni, and Jeremy Sugarman (New York: Oxford University Press, 1998), pp. 67–87.

18. Institute of Medicine, *Women and Health Research* (Washington, DC: National Academy Press, 1994), p. 43.

19. Sandra Harding, "Women, Science, and Society," *Science* 281 (1998): 1599–1600.

20. Food and Drug Administration, "Guideline for the Study and Evaluation of Gender Differences in the Clinical Evaluation of Drugs," *Federal Register* 58 (1993): 39,406–39, 411.

21. National Institutes of Health, "NIH Guidelines on the Inclusion of Women and Minorities as Subjects in Clinical Research," *Federal Register* 59 (1994): 14,508–14, 513.

22. Food and Drug Administration, "Regulations Requiring Manufacturers to Assess the Safety and Effectiveness of New Drugs and Biological Products in Pediatric Patients," *Federal Register* 63 (1998): 66,632–66, 638; National Institutes of Health, "NIH Policy and Guidelines on the Inclusion of Children as Participants in Research Involving Human Subjects," 1998. Accessible on the Internet at http://www.nih.gov/grants/guide/notice-files/not98–024.html.

23. Food and Drug Administration, "Investigational New Drug Applications and New Drug Applications," *Federal Register* 63 (1998): 6854–6862.

24. W. Wayt Gibbons, "What Are Obstacles to Ideal Care?" *Scientific American,* September 1996, 166.

25. Food and Drug Modernization Act, U.S. Code, vol. 42, § 282 (j) (1999 Supplement).

26. National Institutes of Health Council of Public Representatives, "Council Meeting Summary Minutes," 21 April 1999. Accessible on the Internet at http://www.nih.gov/welcome/publicliaison/.

27. Stephanie Stapleton, "Is Best Cancer Care Available?" *AMA News,* 3 August 1998, 5.

28. National Cancer Institute, "Agreement between the National Institutes of Health and the American Association of Health Plans in Support of Clinical Trials," 1999. Accessible on the Internet at http://cancertrials.nci.nih.gov.

29. Sharona Hoffman, "A Proposal for Federal Legislation to Address Health Insurance Coverage for Experimental and Investigational Treatments," *Oregon Law Review* 78 (1999): 203–273. See also National Cancer Institute, "Legislation and Insurance Coverage," 2000. Accessible on the Internet at http:///www.cancertrials.nci. nih.gov/news/coverage/index.html.

30. White House Office of the Press Secretary, "President Clinton Takes New Action to Encourage Participation in Clinical Trials," 7 June 2000. Accessible on the Internet at http://www.whitehouse.gov/WH/New/html/20000607.html.

31. Martin L. Brown, "Cancer Patient Care in Clinical Trials Sponsored by the National Cancer Institute: What Does It Cost?" *Journal of the National Cancer Institute* 91 (1999): 818–819.

32. Leigh Page, "Insurance Coverage for Clinical Trials,"*AMA News*, 23–30 March 1998, 3, 31–32.

33. National Breast Cancer Coalition, "Legislative Priority #3: Insurance Coverage for Routine Patient Care Costs Associated With Participation in Quality Clinical Trials," 1999. Accessible on the Internet at http://www.natlbcc.org/agenda/brief/p3.asp.

34. Harold Edgar and David Rothman, "New Rules for New Drugs: The Challenge of AIDS to the Regulatory Process," *Milbank Quarterly* 68 (suppl. 1, 1990): 111–142.

35. National Commission for the Protection of Human Subjects of Biomedical and Behavioral Research, *The Belmont Report: Ethical Principles and Guidelines for the Protection of Human Subjects of Research* (Washington, DC: Government Printing Office, 1979).

36. Epstein, *Impure Science,* p. 222.

37. Connie Mack, "Lift F.D.A. Roadblock on Experimental Drugs," *New York Times,* 19 February 1995, p. 12.

38. Institute of Medicine, *Women and Health Research*, p. 15.

39. National Cancer Institute, "Restructuring Clinical Trials," 1998. Accessible on the Internet at http://cancertrials.nci.gov/NCI_CANCER_TRIALS/zones/Tools/ Booklets/Plan/intro.html.

40. Spiers, "Community Consultation: Part II," p. 5.

41. Epstein, *Impure Science*, p. 188 (quoting Martin Delaney).

42. Vanessa Merton, "The Exclusion of Pregnant, Pregnable, and Once-Pregnable People (A.K.A. Women) from Biomedical Research," *American Journal of Law & Medicine* 19 (1993): 377–380.

43. Alta Charo, "Protecting Us to Death: Women, Pregnancy, and Clinical Research," *Saint Louis University Law Journal* 38 (1993): 135–167.

44. Rebecca Dresser, "Wanted: Single, White Male for Medical Research," *Hastings Center Report* 22 (January-February 1992): 24–29.

45. "Federal Policy for the Protection of Human Subjects," *Federal Register* 56 (1991): 28,016–28, 017.

46. Samuel Hellman and Deborah S. Hellman, "Of Mice But Not Men: Problems of the Randomized Clinical Trial," *New England Journal of Medicine* 324: (1991) 1585–1589.

47. Advisory Committee on Human Radiation Experiments, *Final Report* (New York: Oxford University Press, 1996).

48. Nancy Kass, et al., "Trust: The Fragile Foundation of Contemporary Biomedical Research," *Hastings Center Report* 26 (September-October 1996): 20–24. A news ac-

count of a fetal tissue transplant trial for Parkinson's disease also highlights deficiencies in patients' understanding. In the trial, some participants were randomly assigned to a placebo control group and underwent "sham" surgical procedures without receiving the tissue. Although they had agreed to participate after being told that they might not receive the tissue, some were chagrined to discover that this actually had occurred. One woman said, "I was crushed." Even though she knew there was a possibility she had not gotten the experimental intervention, she said, "I really thought I had. I thought I couldn't be fooled. But I was." Laura Johannes, "Sham Surgery Is Used to Test Effectiveness of Novel Operations," *Wall Street Journal*, 11 December 1998, A1, A8.

49. Ezekiel Emanuel, "A Phase I Trial on the Ethics of Phase I Trials," *Journal of Clinical Oncology* 13 (1995): 1049–1051.

50. Christopher Daugherty, et al., "Perceptions of Cancer Patients and Their Physicians Involved in Phase I Trials," *Journal of Clinical Oncology* 13 (1995): 1062–1072.

51. Advisory Committee on Human Radiation Experiments, *Final Report*, pp. 713–716. Even the government's clinical trials database contains language that conflates trial participation with receiving proven health care. See Rebecca Dresser, "Surfing for Studies," *Hastings Center Report* 29 (November-December 1999): 26–27.

52. Jeremy Sugarman, et al., "What Patients Say About Medical Research," *IRB: A Review of Human Subjects Research* 20 (July-August 1998): 1–7.

53. Maurie Markman, "The Objective Clinical Scientist Versus the Advocate: A Complex Ethical and Political Dilemma Facing Cancer Investigators and the Public," *Cancer Investigation* 13 (1995): 324–326.

54. Daugherty et al., "Perceptions of Cancer Patients."

55. Sherwin Nuland, "Medicine Isn't Just for the Sick Anymore," *New York Times*, 10 May 1998, §4, p. 1.

56. This topic is discussed in greater detail in chapter 7.

57. Franklin Miller and Andrew Shorr, "Advertising for Clinical Research," *IRB: A Review of Human Subjects Research* 21 (September-October 1999): 1–4.

58. American Cancer Society, "Making Strides Against Breast Cancer," *New York Times Magazine*, 10 October 1999, p. 51.

59. George Annas, "FDA's Compassion for Desperate Drug Companies," *Hastings Center Report* 20 (January-February 1990): 35–37.

60. Spiers, "Community Consultation: Part II," p. 5.

61. Mary Anglin, "From the Inside Out: Implications of Breast Cancer Activism for Biomedical Policies and Practices," *Social Science and Medicine* 44 (1997): 1412.

62. Franz Ingelfinger, "Informed (But Uneducated) Consent," *New England Journal of Medicine* 287 (1972): 465–466.

63. Lisa Eckenwiler, "Attention to Difference and Women's Consent to Research," *IRB: A Review of Human Subjects Research* 20 (November-December 1998): 6–11.

64. Gina Kolata and Kurt Eichenwald, "For the Uninsured, Drug Trials Are Health Care," *New York Times*, 22 June 1999, A1, C11.

65. Sugarman, et al., "What Patients Say," p. 6.

66. Gina Kolata, "Critics Fault Secret Effort to Test AIDS Drug," *New York Times*, 19 September 1989, A21.

67. Alessandra Stanley, "Call It Hope, or Quackery, When Cancer Strikes," *New York Times*, 31 July 1998, A4.

68. Committee on Drugs, "Guidelines for the Ethical Conduct of Studies to Evaluate Drugs in Pediatric Populations," *Pediatrics* 95 (1995): 286–294.

69. Rebecca Dresser, "Mentally Disabled Research Subjects: The Enduring Policy Issues," *Journal of the American Medical Association* 276 (1996): 67–72.

70. Institute of Medicine, *Review of the Fialuridine (FIAU) Clinical Trials* (Washington, DC: National Academy Press, 1995).

71. Robert Oldham, "Patient-Funded Cancer Research," *New England Journal of Medicine* 316 (1987): 46–47.

72. George J. Annas, "Faith (Healing), Hope and Charity at the FDA: The Politics of AIDS Drug Trials," *Villanova Law Review* 34 (1989): 786.

73. Paul D. Stolley, "The Hazards of Misguided Compassion," *Annals of Internal Medicine* 118 (1993): 822–823.

74. Rachel Nowak, "AIDS Researchers, Activists Fight Crisis in Clinical Trials," *Science* 269 (995): 1666–1667.

75. American Society of Clinical Oncology, "Patient Information: Mixed Results in High-Dose Chemotherapy/Bone Marrow Transplant Studies for Women With Breast Cancer," 1999. Accessible on the Internet at http://www.asco.org/people/nr/html/patient/mixedresults.htm.

76. William J. Gradisher, "High-Dose Chemotherapy and Breast Cancer," *Journal of the American Medical Association* 282 (1999): 1378–1380.

77. Richard Saver, "Reimbursing New Technologies: Why Are the Courts Judging Experimental Medicine?" *Stanford Law Review* 44 (1992): 1095–1131.

78. Jonas Burgh, "Where Next With Stem-Cell-Supported High-Dose Therapy for Breast Cancer?" *Lancet* 355 (2000): 944–945. The sole trial suggesting that the experimental procedure was superior to conventional treatment was later discredited because the investigator misrepresented the study data. Raymond Weiss, et al., "High-Dose Chemotherapy for High-Risk Primary Breast Cancer: An On-Site Review of the Bezwoda Study," *Lancet* 355 (2000): 999–1003. High-dose chemotherapy and bone marrow transplantation remain under investigation for women with less advanced disease. NIH News Release, "Don't Write Off High-Dose Chemotherapy With Bone Marrow Transplant for Breast Cancer, Experts Say," 19 May 2000. Accessible on the Internet at http://www.nih.gov/news/pr/may2000/nci-19htm.

79. Lonnie B. Hanauer, "When Advocacy Harms," *New York Times*, 20 March 1999, A26.

80. Elizabeth Shackelford, "Patients Are Victims of the Politics of Cancer," *New York Times,* 22 April 1999, A30.

81. David Eddy, "Investigational Treatments—How Strict Should We Be?" *Journal of the American Medical Association* 278 (1997): 179–185.

82. Temple, "Are Surrogate Markers Adequate?" pp. 792–793.

83. Nowak, "AIDS Researchers, Activists Fight Crisis," p. 1667 (quoting Peter Staley).

84. Gina Kolata, "Debate Reopens on AIDS Access," *New York Times,* 12 September 1994, A16.

85. Ibid.

86. Epstein, *Impure Science*, pp. 315–316.

87. Larry Churchill, et al., "Genetic Research as Therapy: Implications of 'Gene Therapy' for Informed Consent," *Journal of Law, Medicine & Ethics* 26 (1998): 38–47.

88. Shulman and Brown, "Food and Drug Administration's Early Access Initiatives," p. 505.

89. Kolata and Eichenwald, "For the Uninsured, Drug Trials Are Health Care," C11.

90. Larry Kramer, "A Good News/Bad News AIDS Joke," *New York Times Magazine*, 14 July 1996, 27.

91. Anglin, "From the Inside Out," p. 1412.

92. National Breast Cancer Coalition, "Legislative Priority #3: Insurance Coverage."

93. Dresser, "Surfing for Studies," p. 27.

94. G. Marie Swanson and Amy J. Ward, "Recruiting Minorities Into Clinical Trials: Toward a Participant-Friendly System," *Journal of the National Cancer Institute* 87 (1995): 1747–1759.

95. Ibid., p. 1755.

96. Institute of Medicine, *Women and Health Research*, p. 121.

97. John Smith, "Science, Politics, and Policy: The Tacrine Debate," *Food and Drug Law Journal* 47 (1992): 511–532.

98. Ibid., p. 527.

99. David Wasserman, "Self-Help Groups, Affinity-Based Community, and Civil Society," National Commission on Civic Renewal Working Paper #12 (University of Maryland: Institute for Philosophy and Public Policy, n.d.), p. 23.

100. M. J. Friedrich, "Issues in Prostate Cancer Screening," *Journal of the American Medical Association* 281 (1999): 1573–1575. In a story about high-dose chemotherapy and bone marrow transplantation for advanced breast cancer, health reporter Robert Bazell acknowledged the difficulty of being honest. In writing about two friends who had recently died of breast cancer despite undergoing the procedure, Bazell admitted he had not disclosed to them his honest belief that the transplants would probably fail. The reason? "I know that is not what they wanted to hear, and I would not have had the courage to say it." Robert Bazell, "Growth Industry," *New Republic*, 15 March 1993, 13–14. In chapter 8, I argue that advocates owe it to constituents to speak frankly about the prospect of receiving a direct health benefit from unproven interventions.

101. Sandra Oliver, "How Can Health Service Users Contribute to the NHS Research and Development Programmes?" *British Medical Journal* 310 (1995): 1318–1320. Indeed, it is becoming more common for advocacy groups to help researchers recruit study participants. For an example, see NIH News Release, "NIAMS Funds the North American Spondylitis Consortium," 27 September 1999. Accessible on the Internet at http://www.nih.gov/niams/news/niams-27.htm.

102. Richard A. Deyo, et al., "The Messenger Under Attack—Intimidation of Researchers By Special-Interest Groups," *New England Journal of Medicine* 336 (1997): 1176–1180.

103. Comprehensive Working Group on Informed Consent in Cancer Clinical Trials, "Recommendations of the Development of Informed Consent Documents for Cancer Clinical Trials," 1998. Accessible on the Internet at http://cancertrials.nci.nih.gov/NCI_CANCER_TRIALS/zones/TrialInfo/Deciding/InformedConsent/recom.html.

104. Laurie Flynn, "Research and Ethics Must Go Hand in Hand," *The Decade of the Brain: A NAMI Publication* 9, no. 3 (1999): 1.

105. Christine Brunswick, "Statement to IOM Committee on Reimbursement of Routine Patient Care Costs for Medicare," 24 March 1999. Accessible on the Internet at http://www.natlbcc.org/agenda/testimony/trialschristine.asp.

106. Patty Delaney, "The FDA: What Does It Do For Cancer Patients?" 1997. Accessible at the Internet at http://www.fda.gov/oashi/cancer/pdpaat.html.

107. Hazel Thornton, "Alliance Between Medical Professionals and Consumers Already Exists in Breast Cancer," *British Medical Journal* 316 (1998): 148.

108. Gina Kolata, "Critics Fault Secret Effort to Test AIDS Drug," *New York Times*, 19 September 1989, A21.

109. Chapter 7 discusses this topic in detail.

110. Drummond Rennie, "Fair Conduct and Fair Reporting of Clinical Trials," *Journal of the American Medical Association* 282 (1999): 1766–1768.

111. Kass et al., "Trust: The Fragile Foundation," p. 28.

112. Flynn, "Research and Ethics," p. 1. Another example is the National Breast Cancer Coalition's press release issued after an audit found ethics violations in a trial evaluating high-dose chemotherapy and bone marrow transplantation for breast cancer. The release quoted the coalition's president, Fran Visco, as follows: "this trial clearly shows the need for and importance of consumer advocacy in the research process. In the future, we need to make certain that women have the appropriate scientific evidence and comprehensive information about how the trial will be run before consenting to participate." National Breast Cancer Coalition, "For Immediate Release," 4 February 2000. Accessible on the Internet at http://www.nbcc.org/press/Bonemarrow.asp.

113. Matthew C. Lovell, "Second Thoughts: Do the FDA's Responses to a Fatal Drug Trial and the AIDS Activist Community's Doubts About Early Access to Drugs Hint at a Shift in Basic FDA Policy?" *Food and Drug Law Journal* 51 (1996): 273–294.

114. Karen Stabiner, *To Dance With the Devil: The New War on Breast Cancer* (New York: Dell Publishing, 1997), p. 124.

115. Denise Grady, "Breast Cancer Studies Stir Doubts On a Drugs-Transplant Therapy," *New York Times*, 16 April 1999, A1.

116. Epstein, *Impure Science*, p. 345 (italics in original).

117. National Breast Cancer Coalition, "Legislative Activities," 1999. Accessible on the Internet at http://www.natlbcc.org/legintro.asp.

118. Kolata and Eichenwald, "For the Uninsured, Drug Trials Are Health Care," C11.

119. Katherine Rich, "Close to the Bone," *New York Times Magazine*, 19 December 1999, 102.

120. Daniel Callahan, *False Hopes: Why America's Quest for Perfect Health Is a Recipe for Failure* (New York: Simon and Schuster, 1998).

Chapter 4

1. Sheryl Gay Stolberg, "In 'Mother Teresa's Waiting Room,' Optimism," *New York Times*, 14 April 1999, A16.

2. Claude Barfield and Bruce Smith, "Introduction," in *The Future of Biomedical Research*, ed. Claude Barfield and Bruce Smith (Washington, DC: American Enterprise Institute, 1997), p. 2.

3. Institute of Medicine, *Scientific Opportunities and Public Needs* (Washington DC: National Academy Press, 1998), pp. 56–57.

4. Christopher Anderson, "Research and Health Care Costs," *Science* 261(1993): 416–418.

5. Peter Neumann and Eileen Sandberg, "Trends in Health Care R & D and Technology Innovation," *Health Affairs* 17 (1998): 111–119.

6. Robert Levine, "The Impact of HIV Infection on Society's Perception of Clinical Trials," *Kennedy Institute of Ethics Journal* 4 (1994): 93–98.

7. Rebecca Dresser, "Setting Priorities for Science Support," *Hastings Center Report* 28 (May-June 1998): 21–23.

8. NIH Working Group on Priority Setting, *Setting Research Priorities at the National Institutes of Health*, NIH Publication No. 97–4265 (Washington, DC, 1997).

9. Institute of Medicine, *Scientific Opportunities*.

10. Daniel Callahan, "Shaping Biomedical Research Priorities: The Case of the National Institutes of Health," *Health Policy Analysis* 7 (1999): 123.

11. Roger B. Dworkin, *Limits: The Role of the Law in Bioethical Decision Making* (Bloomington, Indiana: Indiana University Press, 1996), pp. 146–147.

12. John F. Lauerman, "Turning the Tables," *Harvard Magazine*, July-August 1998, 26–28.

13. James Fallows, "The Political Scientist," *New Yorker*, 7 June 1999, 68.

14. NIH Working Group, *Setting Research Priorities*, p. 4.

15. Ibid., p. 8.

16. Ibid., p. 9.

17. Harold E. Varmus, "The View from the National Institutes of Health," in *Future of Biomedical Research*, ed. Barfield and Smith, p. 15.

18. Ibid.

19. Ibid.

20. Institute of Medicine, *Scientific Opportunities*, p. 20.

21. For example, though its relevance to human disease was initially unclear, basic science research on recombinant DNA produced knowledge that enabled scientists to produce synthetic growth hormone and other genetically engineered drugs. NIH Working Group, *Setting Research Priorities*, p. 9.

22. Institute of Medicine, *Scientific Opportunities*, p. 20.

23. For example, it was discovered that a gene linked to breast cancer in mice also affected brain tissue development. NIH Working Group, *Setting Research Priorities*, p. 3.

24. Ibid.

25. Ibid., pp. 11–13, 15.

26. Institute of Medicine, *Scientific Opportunities*, p. 27.

27. Senate Labor and Human Resources Committee, Subcommittee on Public Health and Safety, *Biomedical Research Priorities: Who Should Decide?* 105th Cong. 1st Sess., 1 May 1997, 76–78.

28. Ibid.

29. Judith A. Johnson, *Disease Funding and NIH Priority Setting*, Congressional Research Service Report 97–917 (26 March 1998), 5.

30. Institute of Medicine, *Scientific Opportunities*, p. 33.

31. Ibid.

32. Senate Labor, Health and Human Services and Education Subcommittee, Committee on Appropriations, *Statement of Harold Varmus*, 106th Congress, 1st sess., 6 May 1999. Accessible on the Internet at http://www.senate.gov/appropriations/labor/vrms5_6.htm.

33. Tammy O. Tengs, "Planning for Serendipity: A New Strategy to Prosper from Health Research," Progressive Policy Institute Health Priorities Project Policy Report No. 2, July 1998, 3.

34. Ibid., pp. 2, 9.

35. Callahan, "Shaping Biomedical Research Priorities," p. 126.

36. Daniel Callahan, *False Hopes: Why America's Quest for Perfect Health Is a Recipe for Disaster* (New York: Simon and Schuster, 1998).

37. Senate Labor and Human Resources Committee, *Biomedical Research Priorities*, p. 42.

38. Judith Randal, "How to Divvy Up NIH's Research Pie Sparks Debate," *Journal of the National Cancer Institute* 91 (1999): 411.

39. Sheryl Stolberg, "Childhood Cancer Patients Find Survival Has Price," *New York Times*, 3 January 1999, A1.

40. Joan Stephenson, "US AIDS Research Office Chief: Intensify Vaccine, Prevention Research," *Journal of the American Medical Association* 280 (1998): 1211–1213.

41. Susan Sachs, "Public Clamor Puts Focus on 'Clusters' in Cancer Research," *New York Times,* 21 September 1998, A1.

42. J. A. Weintraub, "Maternal and Child Oral Health Issues: Research," *Journal of Public Health Dentistry* 50 (1990): 447–455.

43. Elizabeth Pennisi, "Academic Sequencers Challenge Celera in a Sprint to the Finish," *Science* 283 (1999): 1822–1823.

44. Carolyn M. Clancy and John M. Eisenberg, "Outcomes Research: Measuring the End Results of Health Care," *Science* 282 (1998): 245–246.

45. Institute of Medicine, *The Unequal Burden of Cancer: An Assessment of NIH Research and Programs for Ethnic Minorities and the Medically Underserved* (Washington, DC: National Academy Press, 1999).

46. "Research Funding for Child and Adolescent Mental Disorders Falls Well Below Goals in National Plan," *Psychiatric Services* 46 (1995): 418.

47. Norman Daniels and James Sabin, "Limits to Health Care: Fair Procedures, Democratic Deliberation, and the Legitimacy Problem for Insurers," *Philosophy and Public Affairs* 26 (1997): 303–350, 319.

48. Ibid., p. 321.

49. Ibid.

50. William B. Rizzo, "Lorenzo's Oil—Hope and Disappointment," *New England Journal of Medicine* 329 (1993): 801–802.

51. Marcia Angell, "Caring for Women's Health—What Is the Problem?" *New England Journal of Medicine* 329 (1993): 271–272.

52. Rebecca Dresser, "Funds for Research on Conditions Primarily Affecting Women: What Is a Fair Share?" *Journal of Gender-Specific Medicine* 2 (September-October 1999): 23–26.

53. Neumann and Sandberg, "Trends in Health Care R & D," pp. 117–118.

54. Institute of Medicine, *Scientific Opportunities*, p. 33.

55. Cary P. Gross, Gerard F. Anderson, and Neil R. Powe, "The Relation Between Funding By the National Institutes of Health and the Burden of Disease," *New England Journal of Medicine* 340 (1999): 1881–1887.

56. Ibid., p. 1886.

57. Ibid, p. 1885.

58. Ibid.

59. According to Daniels and Sabin, members of some European national commissions that were asked to set health care priorities report that the consensus-based abstract principles they initially adopted were too vague to provide meaningful or acceptable resolutions when applied in practice. The groups are now focused on devising fair procedures to govern specific decisions. Daniels and Sabin, "Limits to Health Care," p. 349.

60. Council on Ethical and Judicial Affairs, American Medical Association, "Ethical

Issues in Health Care System Reform," *Journal of the American Medical Association* 272 (1994): 1059–1062.

61. Daniels and Sabin, "Limits to Health Care," p. 321.

62. ABCNEWS.com, "Rehnquist Speaks," 12 February 1999. Accessible on the Internet at http://204.202.137.114/sections/us/PoliticalNation/rehnquist990212.html.

63. Tom R. Tyler, *Why People Obey the Law* (New Haven: Yale University Press, 1990).

64. Ibid., p. 137.

65. Ibid.

66. Ibid., p. 107.

67. Daniels and Sabin, "Limits to Health Care," p. 327.

68. Ibid., p. 330.

69. Ibid., p. 340.

70. Ibid., p. 323. As Daniels and Sabin note, the features they believe are important to a fair allocation system resemble principles on deliberative democratic decision making proposed by Amy Gutmann and Dennis Thompson, which are discussed in chapter 5. Amy Gutmann and Dennis Thompson, *Democracy and Disagreement* (Cambridge, Massachusetts: Harvard University Press, 1996).

71. Guido Calabresi and Philip Bobbitt, *Tragic Choices* (New York: W. W. Norton and Company, 1978).

72. Daniels and Sabin, "Limit to Health Care," pp. 313–314.

73. Tengs, "Planning for Serendipity," p. 2.

74. Paul Menzel, et al., "Toward a Broader View of Values in Cost-Effectiveness Analysis of Health," *Hastings Center Report* 29 (May-June, 1999): 7–15.

75. In 1999, the NIH sponsored a workshop to discuss application of disease burden concepts to research priority setting. For discussion, see Office of the NIH Director, "Proceedings of the 79th Meeting of the Advisory Committee to the Director of the National Institutes of Health," 2 December 1999. Accessible on the Internet at http://www.nih.gov/about/director/dec99min.htm.

76. Senate Labor and Human Resources Committee, *Biomedical Research Priorities*, p. 85.

77. Arthur Kornberg, "Support for Basic Biomedical Research: How Breakthroughs Occur," in *Future of Biomedical Research*, ed. Barfield and Smith, p. 38.

78. Tengs, "Planning for Serendipity," p. 2.

79. Floyd E. Bloom, "Priority Setting Quixotic or Essential?" *Science* 282 (1998): 1641.

80. Philip A. Griffiths, "Public Briefing," 17 February 1999. Accessible on the Internet at http://www.nas.edu/new/21de.html. The panel was discussing research agency compliance with the Government Performance and Results Act, which requires all federal agencies to provide to Congress 1) a strategic plan, 2) a performance plan with specific annual targets, and 3) a report on success in meeting those targets. Strategic plans must be revised every three years and performance plans and reports submitted every year. Although not directly aimed at NIH priority setting, this new law will require the NIH to engage in a more systematic approach to funding allocation. Committee on Science, Engineering, and Public Policy, National Academy of Sciences, *Evaluating Federal Research Programs: Research and the Government Performance and Results Act*, 1999. Accessible on the Internet at http://www.nap.edu/readingroom/books/pra/preface.html. The NIH performance plans and reports are accessible on the Internet at http://www.nih.gov/whatsnew.html.

Chapter 5

1. Robert Lipsyte, "It's Enough to Make You Sick, the Way Patients Get Treated," *New York Times,* 21 June 1998, A7.

2. Phil Gunby, "Washington Marchers Unite to Conquer Cancer," *Journal of the American Medical Association* 280 (1998): 1039.

3. Representative David Obey (D-WI), "Appropriations Battle," story by Peter Overby, *Weekend Saturday,* National Public Radio, 26 September 1998.

4. Institute of Medicine, *Scientific Opportunities and Public Needs: Improving Priority Setting at the National Institutes of Health* (Washington, DC: National Academy Press, 1998), p. 13.

5. Bruce Agnew, "Two in a Row: A Whopping Budget Boost for NIH," *Journal of NIH Research* 8 (November 1996): 19–20.

6. Judith Johnson, *Disease Funding and NIH Priority Setting,* Congressional Research Service Report 97–917 (26 March 1998).

7. Eliot Marshall, "Lobbyists Seek to Reslice NIH's Pie," *Science* 276 (1997): 346.

8. Ibid., pp. 344–346.

9. Agnew, "Two in a Row," p. 20.

10. Marshall, "Lobbyists Seek to Reslice NIH's Pie," p. 344.

11. John Lauerman, "Turning the Tables," *Harvard Magazine,* July-August 1998, 26–28; Jocelyn Kaiser, "NIH's Harvest of Special Projects," *Science* 274 (1996): 167.

12. House Appropriations Committee, Subcommittee on Labor, Health and Human Services, and Education, *Appropriations for the National Institutes of Health,* 105th Cong., 1st sess., 10 June 1997.

13. Agnew, "Two in a Row," p. 19.

14. Rebecca Dresser, "Setting Priorities for Science Support," *Hastings Center Report* 28 (May-June 1998): 21–23.

15. Senate Labor and Human Resources Committee, Subcommittee on Public Health and Safety, *Biomedical Health Priorities: Who Should Decide?* 105th Cong., 1st sess., 1 May 1997.

16. Institute of Medicine, *Scientific Opportunities,* p. 57.

17. Ibid., pp. 61–66

18. Ibid., p. 62

19. Ibid., p. 64.

20. Ibid., p. 70.

21. House Committee, *Appropriations,* p. 2492.

22. Timothy Murphy, "No Time for an AIDS Backlash," *Hastings Center Report* 21 (March-April 1991): 7–11.

23. Rebecca Dresser, "Wanted: Single White Male for Medical Research," *Hastings Center Report* 22 (January-February 1992): 24–29.

24. Daniel Sarewitz, "Social Change and Science Policy," *Issues in Science and Technology,* Summer 1997, 29–32.

25. "Funding Priorities, Peer Review: An Interview with Harold Varmus," *Journal of NIH Research* 9 (August 1997): 21–25.

26. Marshall, "Lobbyists Seek to Reslice NIH's Pie," p. 346.

27. Mary K. Anglin, "Working from the Inside Out: Implications of Breast Cancer Activism for Biomedical Policies and Practices," *Social Science and Medicine* 44 (1996): 1403–1415.

28. Amy Langer, "The Role of Advocacy in Cancer Research: Not a Monster," *Cancer Investigation* 15 (1997): 500–502.

29. Institute of Medicine, *Approaching Death: Improving Care at the End of Life* (Washington, DC: National Academy Press, 1997).

30. Institute of Medicine, *Scientific Opportunities*, pp. 54, 72–73.

31. Sarewitz, "Social Change and Science Policy," pp. 30–31.

32. NIH Working Group on Priority Setting, *Setting Research Priorities at the National Institutes of Health,* NIH pub. no. 97–4265 (Washington, DC, 1997).

33. David B. Resnick, *The Ethics of Science: An Introduction* (New York: Routledge, 1998).

34. Stephanie Stapleton, "Lobby for Labs: Biomed Research Campaigning for Funding Increase," *AMA News,* 9 February 1998, 1, 29.

35. Sheryl Stolberg, "New Challenge to Idea That 'AIDS is Special,'" *New York Times*, 12 November 1997, A1, A18; Murphy, "No Time for an AIDS Backlash," pp. 7–8.

36. Institute of Medicine, *Scientific Opportunities*, pp. 54–55.

37. Institute of Medicine, *Scientific Opportunities*, p. 56.

38. Daniel Callahan, *False Hopes: Why America's Quest for Perfect Health is a Recipe for Failure* (New York: Simon and Schuster, 1998).

39. Institute of Medicine, *Approaching Death*, p. 255.

40. Johnson, *Disease Funding and NIH Priority Setting*, p. 1. This tendency continued into the next decade as well. See Andrew Lawler, "NIH Headed for Big Boost, Others Struggle," *Science* 288 (2000): 1155.

41. "Medical Research Funding," *New York Times*, 6 January 1998, A20.

42. Harold E. Varmus, "The View from the National Institutes of Health," in *The Future of Biomedical Research*, ed. Claude Barfield and Bruce Smith (Washington, DC: American Enterprise Institute, 1997), pp. 9–15, 14.

43. Buford Rolin, Chairman, Indian Health Board, speaking at Senate Committee on Indian Affairs, *Hearing on Unmet Indian Health Needs*, 21 May 1998, LEXIS, Federal Document Clearing House Congressional Testimony.

44. Tom R. Tyler, *Why People Obey the Law* (New Haven: Yale University Press, 1990).

45. Norman Daniels and James Sabin, "Limits to Health Care: Fair Procedures, Democratic Deliberation, and the Legitimacy Problem for Insurers," *Philosophy and Public Affairs* 26 (1997): 303–350.

46. Amy Gutmann and Dennis Thompson, *Democracy and Disagreement* (Cambridge, Massachusetts: Harvard University Press, 1996), p. 12.

47. Amy Gutmann and Dennis Thompson, "Deliberating about Bioethics," *Hastings Center Report* 27 (May-June 1997): 38–41.

48. Gutmann and Thompson, *Democracy and Disagreement*, pp. 152–164.

49. Gutmann and Thompson, "Deliberating About Bioethics," p. 39.

50. Ibid., pp. 39–41.

51. Gutmann and Thompson, *Democracy and Disagreement*, pp. 199–229.

52. Council of Public Representatives, "Meeting Minutes," 21 April 1999. Accessible on the Internet at http://www.nih.gov/about/publicliaison/042199minutes.htm.

53. Carla Garnett, "COPR Provides New Forum for Interacting with Public," *NIH Record*, 18 May 1999, 1, 6–7.

54. NIH Office of Communications and Public Liaison, 2000. Accessible on the Internet at http://www.nih.gov/od/ocpl.

55. Harold E. Varmus, "Fiscal Year 2000 President's Budget Request for the Na-

tional Institutes of Health," 22 February 1999. Accessible on the Internet at http:// www.nih.gov/about/director/022299.htm.

56. Institute of Medicine, *Scientific Opportunities*, p. 68.

57. NIH Director, "Call for Nominations for Membership on the NIH Director's Council of Public Representatives," 1998. Accessible on the Internet at http:// www.nih.gov/about/publicliaison/COPRnomination.htm.

58. NIH Director, "Call for Nominations," pp. 1–2.

59. The call for nominations produced 250 submissions. Twenty applicants were chosen for the council, and the remaining were designated "COPR Associates" assigned to comment on council activities and participate in other NIH groups. Garnett, "COPR Provides New Forum," p. 6.

60. Institute of Medicine, *Scientific Opportunities*, p. 57.

61. Ibid., p. 65.

62. Director's Council of Public Representatives, "Membership Roster," 1999. Accessible on the Internet at http://www.nih.gov/about/publicliaison/COPRroster.htm.

63. NIH Director, "Call for Nominations," p. 1.

64. David Dickson, *The New Politics of Science* (Chicago: University of Chicago Press, 1988), p. 257.

65. Langer, "The Role of Advocacy in Cancer Research," p. 501.

66. Richard Sclove, *Democracy and Technology* (New York: Guilford Press, 1995), p. 192.

67. NIH Working Group on Priority Setting, *Setting Research Priorities*, p. 3.

68. Varmus, "View from the National Institutes of Health," p. 13.

69. *Codes of Professional Responsibility*, 3d ed., Rena A. Gorlin, ed. (Washington, DC: Bureau of National Affairs, 1994), p. 619.

70. Ibid.

71. NIH Director, "Call for Nominations," p. 2.

72. William Brinkley, Jeremy Wood, and Howard H. Garrison, "Increased Funding for NIH: A Biomedical Science Perspective," *FASEB Journal* 12 (1998): 1431–1435.

73. NIH Working Group on Priority Setting, "Setting Research Priorities," p. 3.

74. In a 1999 presentation on public participation, the director of the National Institute of Neurological Disorders and Stroke reported that advocates for numerous organizations were able to work together on developing and refining the institute's strategic research plan. Council of Public Representatives, "Meeting Minutes," 21 April 1999.

Chapter 6

1. Lisa Eckenwiler, "Pursuing Reform in Clinical Research: Lessons from Women's Experience," *Journal of Law, Medicine & Ethics* 27 (1999): 158–170.

2. Paul A. Lombardo, "New Faces on the IRB: Who Speaks for Subjects?" *BioLaw* (1999 Suppl.):428–431.

3. Herbert Spiers, "Community Consultation and AIDS Clinical Trials: Part III," *IRB: A Review of Human Subjects Research* 13 (September-October 1991), 4.

4. David Rothman, *Strangers at the Bedside* (New York: Basic Books, 1991).

5. Robert Veatch, "Human Experimentation Committees: Professional or Representative?" *Hastings Center Report* 5 (October 1975): 31–40.

6. Jay Katz, *Experimentation with Human Beings* (New York: Russell Sage Foun-

dation, 1972), pp. 886–889 (citing U.S. Public Health Service, Protection of the Individual as a Research Subject).

7. National Commission for the Protection of Human Subjects of Biomedical and Behavioral Research, *Report and Recommendations: Institutional Review Boards*, DHEW Publication No. (OS) 78–0008 (Washington, DC: Government Printing Office, 1978), p. 14.

8. Federal Policy for the Protection of Human Subjects, *Federal Register* 56 (1991): 28,015.

9. Federal Policy for the Protection of Human Subjects, 28,014–15. Two other U.S. policies require direct representation of prospective participants. In 1978, the Department of Health and Human Services issued rules governing federally sponsored research involving prisoners. The rules require IRBs that review this category of research to have at least one member who is a prisoner or prisoner representative. Department of Health and Human Services, "Additional Protections Pertaining to Biomedical and Behavioral Research Involving Prisoners as Subjects," *Federal Register* 43 (1978): 53,655. The Department of Education requires that IRBs reviewing certain research involving disabled persons include at least one member "primarily concerned with the welfare of these research subjects." Department of Education, "Disability and Rehabilitation Research: Research Fellowships," *Code of Federal Regulations* 34 (1999): § 356.3(c)(2).

10. Food and Drug Administration, "Protection of Human Subjects; Informed Consent," *Federal Register* 61 (1996): 51,498–51,533.

11. Ibid., p. 51,528.

12. Council for International Organizations of Medical Sciences, *International Ethical Guidelines for Biomedical Research Involving Human Subjects* (Geneva: CIOMS, 1993).

13. Ibid., p. 40.

14. Council for International Organizations of Medical Sciences, *International Guidelines for Ethical Review of Epidemiological Studies*. Reprinted in *Law, Medicine & Health Care* 19 (1991): 247–258.

15. Sally Lehrman, "Jewish Leaders Seek Genetic Guidelines," *Nature* 389 (1997): 322.

16. Vida Foubister, "Research Reservations," *American Medical News*, 31 January 2000, 8–10.

17. Partly in response to this argument, the National Bioethics Advisory Commission recommended that scientists who conduct research using stored tissue samples consult representatives of at-risk groups before proceeding with the research. National Bioethics Advisory Commission, *Research Involving Human Biological Materials: Ethical Issues and Policy Guidance: Report and Recommendations* (Rockville, Maryland: National Bioethics Advisory Commission, 1999), p. 73. The demand for community involvement also extends to other types of research that could have negative social consequences for members of particular groups. Charles Weijer, Gary Goldsand, and Ezekiel Emanuel, "Protecting Communities in Research: Current Guidelines and Limits of Extrapolation," *Nature Genetics* 23 (1999): 275–280.

18. Animal Welfare Act, U. S. Code, vol. 7,§ 2143(b)(1)(B)(iii) (1994).

19. U.S. Congress, Office of Technology Assessment, *Biomedical Ethics in U.S. Public Policy*, OTA-BP-BBS-105 (Washington, DC: U.S. Government Printing Office, 1993).

20. President William J. Clinton, Executive Order 13,137, § 2 (1999). Accessible on the Internet at http://bioethics.gov/nbac_extended.html.

21. Paul M. McNeill, *The Ethics and Politics of Human Experimentation* (New York: Cambridge University Press, 1993), pp. 69–81, 100–104.

22. Jane Gregory and Steve Miller, *Science in Public: Communication, Culture, and Credibility* (New York: Plenum Press, 1998), pp. 235–237.

23. Veatch, "Human Experimentation Committees," p. 36.

24. William J. Curran, "Government Regulation of the Use of Human Subjects in Medical Research: The Approach of Two Federal Agencies," *Daedalus* 98 (1969): 542–594.

25. Tri-Council Policy Statement, "Ethical Conduct of Research Involving Humans: Research Ethics Boards," 1998. Accessible on the Internet at http://www.mrc.gc.ca/ethics/english/index.htm.

26. National Commission for the Protection of Human Subjects, *Report and Recommendations*, p. 14.

27. Mark S. Frankel, "The Development of Policy Guidelines Governing Human Experimentation in the United States: A Case Study of Public Policy-Making for Science and Technology," *Ethics in Science and Medicine* 2 (1975): 43–59.

28. National Commission for the Protection of Human Subjects, *Report and Recommendations*, pp. 1–2.

29. Joan P. Porter, "How Unaffiliated/Nonscientist Members of Institutional Review Boards See Their Roles," *IRB: A Review of Human Subjects Research* 9 (November-December 1987): 1–6.

30. Arlene M. Davis, "Exception from Informed Consent for Emergency Research: Drawing on Existing Skills and Experience," *IRB: A Review of Human Subjects Research* 20 (September-October 1998): 1–8.

31. Annette Dula, "Bearing the Brunt of the New Regulations: Minority Populations," *Hastings Center Report* 27 (January-February 1997): 11–12.

32. President's Commission for the Study of Ethical Problems in Medicine and Biomedical and Behavioral Research, *Implementing Human Research Regulations* (Washington, DC: Government Printing Office, 1983), p. 48.

33. Veatch, "Human Experimentation Committees," p. 37.

34. President's Commission, *Implementing Human Research Regulations*, p. 46.

35. Porter, "How Unaffiliated/Nonscientist Members See Their Roles," p. 2.

36. Tri-Council Policy Statement, "Ethical Conduct of Research."

37. Porter, "How Unaffiliated/Nonscientist Members See Their Roles," p. 2.

38. Rebecca Dresser, "Community Representatives and Nonscientists on the IACUC: What Difference Should It Make?" *ILAR Journal* 40, no. 1 (1999): 29–33.

39. Joan P. Porter, "What Are the Ideal Characteristics of Unaffiliated/Nonscientist IRB Members?" *IRB: A Review of Human Subjects Research* 8 (May-June 1986): 1–6.

40. Ibid., p. 4.

41. Porter, "How Unaffiliated/Nonscientist Members See Their Roles," p. 2.

42. Carol Levine, Nancy N. Dubler, and Robert J. Levine, "Building a New Consensus: Ethical Principles and Policies for Clinical Research on HIV/AIDS," *IRB: A Review of Human Subjects Research* 13 (January-April 1991): 1–17.

43. House Committee on Government Reform and Oversight, Subcommittee on Human Resources, *Oversight of NIH and FDA: Bioethics and the Adequacy of Informed Consent*, 105th Cong. 1st Sess., 8 May 1997, 198–207.

44. McNeill, *Ethics and Politics*, pp. 194–199.

45. Frankel, "Development of Policy Guidelines," p. 51 (citing letter from James Shannon to U.S. Surgeon General).

46. Bernard Barber, et al., *Research on Human Subjects* (New York: Russell Sage Foundation, 1973), p. 197.

47. U.S. Congress, *Biomedical Ethics*, pp. 10, 13.

48. Food and Drug Administration, "Protection of Human Subjects," pp. 51, 515.

49. Ibid., p. 51,516.

50. Davis, "Exception from Informed Consent," p. 4.

51. McNeill, *Ethics and Politics*, pp. 198–199.

52. Veatch, "Human Experimentation Committees," p. 37.

53. Ibid.

54. Department of Health and Human Services Office of Inspector General, *Institutional Review Boards: A Time for Reform*, OEI-01-97-00193 (Washington, DC: Government Printing Office, 1998), p. 8.

55. House Committee on Government Reform and Oversight, *Institutional Review Boards: A System in Jeopardy*, 105th Cong., 2d Sess., 1998. Statement of Robert J. Levine, accessible on the Internet at http://www.house.gov/reform/hr/hearings/hr61198/levine.html.

56. Bartolo, "Tales of Informed Consent: Four Years on an Institutional Review Board," *Health Matrix: Journal of Law-Medicine* 2 (1992): 201.

57. McNeill, *Ethics and Politics*, p. 93.

58. National Commission for the Protection of Human Subjects of Biomedical and Behavioral Research, *Appendix to Report and Recommendations: Institutional Review Boards*, DHEW Publication No. (OS)78–0009 (Washington, DC: Government Printing Office, 1977), pp. 1–31.

59. Porter, "What Are the Ideal Characteristics?" p. 6.

60. McNeill, *Ethics and Politics*, pp. 88–91.

61. Ibid., p. 91.

62. Porter, "What Are the Ideal Characteristics?" p. 6.

63. Department of Health and Human Services Office of Inspector General, *Institutional Review Boards*, p. 18.

64. President's Commission, *Implementing Human Research Regulations*, p. 46.

65. Department of Health and Human Services Office of Inspector General, *Institutional Review Boards*, pp. 17–18.

66. Porter, "What Are the Ideal Characteristics?" p. 6.

67. McNeill, *Ethics and Politics*, pp. 195–196.

68. Ibid., pp. 139–206.

69. Ibid., pp. 194–198.

70. Ibid, pp. 198–199. See also Beverly Woodward, "Challenges to Human Subjects Protections in U.S. Medical Research," *Journal of the American Medical Association* 282 (1999):1947–1952.

71. Department of Health and Human Services Office of Inspector General, *Institutional Review Boards*, p. 1.

72. Ibid., p. 18.

73. Harold Edgar and David J. Rothman, "The Institutional Review Board and Beyond: Future Challenges to the Ethics of Human Experimentation," *Milbank Quarterly* 73 (1995): 489–506.

74. One such exception is an IRB associated with New York City's Community Research Initiative, a research program founded by the People with AIDS Coalition. This IRB played an active and influential part in shaping studies funded by the program. It stands as an example of advocacy success in enhancing the public role in research ethics review. For a description of the committee's work, see Vanessa

Merton, "Community-Based AIDS Research," *Evaluation Review* 14 (1990): 502–537.

75. At a 1997 meeting, an FDA official reported that some investigators and institutions had attempted to meet the emergency research community consultation requirement simply by placing a newspaper advertisement about an upcoming study. Charles Marwick, "Assessment of Exception to Informed Consent," *Journal of the American Medical Association* 278 (1997): 1392–1993.

76. Davis, "Exception from Informed Consent," p. 5. This concern raises representation issues similar to those discussed in chapter 2.

77. Robert J. Levine, "The Institutional Review Board," in *Ethics and Epidemiology*, ed. Steven S. Coughlin and Tom L. Beauchamp (New York: Oxford University Press, 1996) pp. 257–273.

78. Ibid., p. 262.

79. George J. Annas, "Ethics Committees: From Ethical Comfort to Ethical Cover," *Hastings Center Report* 21 (May-June 1991): 18–21.

80. For example, Paul McNeill proposed revising the system to require an equal number of unaffiliated public members and researchers on review committees and establish a new role of research participant representative for public members. McNeill, *Ethics and Politics*, pp. 207–214. Although I believe his proposal has substantial merit, it would demand major changes in policy and practice and thus would face significant political barriers in the United States.

81. Some committees already provide payment to their public members. Robert J. Levine, *Ethics and Regulation of Clinical Research*, 2d ed. (New Haven: Yale University Press, 1986), p. 330.

Chapter 7

1. Susan Love, "Wondering About a Wonder Drug," *New York Times*, 3 August 1999, A19.

2. Timothy Johnson, "Shattuck Lecture—Medicine and the Media," *New England Journal of Medicine* 339 (1998): 87–92.

3. Victor Cohn, "Vaccines and Risks," *Journal of the American Medical Association* 276 (1996): 1917–1918.

4. In 1997, Roper conducted a national survey of 2,256 adults to assess their reliance on the media for health information. When respondents were asked about their primary sources for such information, 40 percent named television, while only 36 percent listed physicians. Many also listed magazines and newspapers as primary sources. National Health Council, *21st Century Housecall: The Link Between Medicine and the Media* (Washington, DC, 1997).

5. Marcia Angell and Jerome Kassirer, "Clinical Research—What Should the Public Believe?" *New England Journal of Medicine* 331 (1994): 189–90.

6. National Cancer Institute Director's Consumer Liaison Group, "Meeting Summary," 17 December 1997. Accessible on the Internet at http://deainfo.nci.nih.gov/ADVISORY/dclg/17dec97.htm.

7. Office of Cancer Communications, National Cancer Institute, *The Public's Perception of Medical and Cancer Research* (Bethesda, Maryland, September 1997), p. 10.

8. Gina Kolata, "A Cautious Awe Greets Drugs That Eradicate Tumors in Mice," *New York Times*, 3 May 1998, A1, A20.

9. Joe Nicholson, "Did the *New York Times* Get It Wrong About Cancer?" *Editor and Publisher,* 30 May 1998, 13–15.

10. Christine Gorman, "The Hope and the Hype," *Time,* 18 May 1998, 38–44.

11. Michael Shapiro, "Pushing the 'Cure': Where a Big Cancer Story Went Wrong," *Columbia Journalism Review,* July-August 1998, 15–16.

12. Gorman, "Hope and Hype," p. 41.

13. Marlene Cimons, Josh Gitlin, and Thomas Maugh, "Cancer Drugs Face Long Road From Mice to Men," *Los Angeles Times,* 6 May 1998, A1.

14. Ian Fisher, "In Excitement Over Cancer Drugs, a Caution Over Premature Hopes," *New York Times,* 5 May 1998, A1, A18.

15. Eliot Marshall, "The Roadblocks to Angiogenesis Blockers," *Science* 280 (1998): 997.

16. News and Editorial Staffs, "Breakthrough of the Year,"*Science* 282 (1998): 2161. The first phase of human testing of endostatin began in late 1999. Difficulties in producing angiostatin have delayed testing of that compound. National Cancer Institute, "Angiogenesis Information" (2000). Accessible on the Internet at http://cancertrials.nci.nih.gov/news/angio/index.html. After seven months of testing, one National Cancer Institute official said he had not observed any dramatic benefits from endostatin. Richard Saltus, "Attacking the Root of Cancer," *Boston Globe,* 30 May 2000, E1.

17. Harold Sox, "Benefit and Harm Associated With Screening for Breast Cancer," *New England Journal of Medicine* 338 (1998): 1145–1146.

18. Suzanne Fletcher, "Whither Scientific Deliberation in Health Policy Recommendations?" *New England Journal of Medicine* 336 (1997): 1180–83.

19. National Institutes of Health Consensus Development Panel, "Conference Statement: Breast Cancer Screening for Women Ages 40–49, January 21–23, 1997," *Journal of the National Cancer Institute* 89 (1997): 1015–20.

20. Fletcher, "Whither Scientific Deliberation?" p. 1181.

21. Charles Marwick, "NIH Consensus Panel Spurs Discontent," *Journal of the American Medical Association* 277 (1997): 519–520.

22. Fletcher, "Whither Scientific Deliberation?" p. 1181.

23. Gina Kolata, "Stand on Mammograms Greeted by Outrage," *New York Times,* 23 January 1997, B9–B10.

24. Gary Taubes, "The Breast-Screening Brawl," *Science* 275 (1997): 1056–1059.

25. Marwick, "NIH Consensus Panel," p. 519.

26. "Mammograms for Younger Women," *New York Times,* 30 March 1997, § 4, p. 10.

27. Kolata, "Stand on Mammograms," B10.

28. Jim Hartz and Rick Chappell, *Worlds Apart: How the Distance Between Science and Journalism Threatens America's Future* (Nashville, Tennessee: First Amendment Center, 1998), p. 58.

29. Ibid., pp. 83–87.

30. Ibid., p. 83.

31. Fletcher, "Whither Scientific Deliberation?" p. 1181.

32. Marcia Angell, "Overdosing on Health Risks," *New York Times Magazine,* 4 May 1997, 44–45.

33. Erika Blacksher, "Complicating the Mammography Message," *Hastings Center Report* 27 (March-April 1997): 48.

34. Hartz and Chappell, *Worlds Apart,* p. 13.

35. Tom Wilkie, "Sources in Science: Who Can We Trust?" *Lancet* 347 (1996): 1308–1311.

36. Ian Dreary, Martha Whiteman and F. Fowkes, "Medical Research and the Popular Media," *Lancet* 351 (1998): 1726–27.

37. Vikki Entwhistle, "Reporting Research in Medical Journals and Newspapers," *British Medical Journal* 310 (1995): 920–923.

38. Wilkie, "Sources in Science," pp. 1308–1309.

39. Hartz and Chappell, *Worlds Apart*, p. 27.

40. Miriam Shuchman and Michael Wilkes, "Medical Scientists and Health News Reporting: A Case of Miscommunication," *Annals of Internal Medicine* 126 (1997): 976–982.

41. Vladimir de Semir, "What Is Newsworthy?" *Lancet* 347 (1996): 1063–1066.

42. Jay Winsten, "Science and the Media: The Boundaries of Truth," *Health Affairs* 4 (1985): 5–23.

43. Hartz and Chappell, *Worlds Apart*, pp. 55–59.

44. Wilkie, "Sources in Science," p. 1309.

45. Victor Cohn, "Coping With Statistics," in *A Field Guide for Science Writers*, eds. Deborah Blum and Mary Knudson (New York: Oxford University Press, 1997), p. 106.

46. Entwhistle, "Reporting Research," p. 922.

47. House of Representatives Committee on Science, *Communicating Science and Engineering in a Sound-Bite World*, 105th Cong. 2d Sess., 14 May 1998. Statement of Deborah Blum, accessible on the Internet at http://www.house.gov/science/blum_05–14.htm.

48. Shuchman and Wilkes, "Medical Scientists," pp. 978–979.

49. Tom Reynolds, "Media Coverage of Cancer Risks May Mislead," *Journal of the National Cancer Institute* 85 (1993): 1366–1368.

50. Dreary, Whiteman and Fowkes, "Medical Research," p. 1726.

51. Angell and Kassirer, "Clinical Research," p. 189.

52. Hartz and Chappell, *Worlds Apart*, pp. 58–59.

53. Winsten, "Science and the Media," p. 9.

54. Hartz and Chappell, *Worlds Apart*, pp. 57–58.

55. Ibid., pp. 56–57.

56. Felicity Barringer, "Reporters, Book Deals and Conflicts," *New York Times,* 5 May 1998, A15.

57. Winsten, "Science and the Media," p. 9.

58. Ibid., p. 5.

59. Dorothy Nelkin, *Selling Science: How the Press Covers Science and Technology*, rev. ed. (New York: W. H. Freeman and Company, 1995), pp. 124–143.

60. Ibid.

61. National Cancer Institute, "Scientists' Views on Communicating Cancer Research: Findings from Focus Groups with Extramural Scientists" (Office of Cancer Communications Health Promotion Branch, Bethesda, Maryland, 1998, photocopy).

62. Lita Nelson, "The Rise of Intellectual Property Protection in the American University," *Science* 279 (1998): 1460–1461.

63. Ezekiel Emanuel and Daniel Steiner, "Institutional Conflict of Interest," *New England Journal of Medicine* 332 (1995): 262–267.

64. John Iglehart, "The American Health Care System: Expenditures," *New England Journal of Medicine* 340 (1999): 70–76.

65. Johnson, "Shattuck Lecture," p. 89.

66. Ibid., p. 89.

67. Pia Pini, "Media Wars," *Lancet* 346 (1995): 1681–1683.

68. Shuchman and Wilkes, "Medical Scientists," p. 68.

69. Laurence Altman, "Inside Medical Journals: A Rising Quest for Profits," *New York Times*, 24 August 1999, D7.

70. The potential problems were highlighted in 1999, when the editors of the two most prestigious U.S. medical journals, the *New England Journal of Medicine* and the *Journal of the American Medical Association*, were forced out over disagreements with executives of the journals' parent organizations. Eliot Marshall, "Kassirer Forced Out at *New England Journal*," *Science* 285 (1999): 648–649.

71. Vladimir de Semir, Cristina Ribas, and Gemma Revuelta, "Press Releases of Science Journal Articles and Subsequent Newspaper Stories on the Same Topic," *Journal of the American Medical Association* 280 (1998): 294–295.

72. Laurent Castelluci, "Embargoes Dictate Coverage of Science," *Journal of the National Cancer Institute* 90 (1998): 958–960.

73. Eliot Marshall, "Public Lashings and Blackballing Enforce System Built on Trust," *Science* 282 (1998): 866.

74. International Committee of Medical Journal Editors, "Uniform Requirements for Manuscripts Submitted to Biomedical Journals," 1997. Accessible on the Internet at http://www.thelancet.com/newlancet/any/author/body.uniform1.html.

75. Marcia Angell and Jerome Kassirer, "The Ingelfinger Rule Revisited," *New England Journal of Medicine* 325 (1991): 1371–1373.

76. Eliot Marshall, "Embargoes: Good, Bad, or 'Necessary Evil'?" *Science* 282 (1998): 863.

77. Nelkin, *Selling Science*, p. 167.

78. Mary Woolley, "Populism and Scientific Decision Making," *Science Communication* 20 (1998): 52–55. See also Michael Crichton, "Ritual Abuse, Hot Air, and Missed Opportunities," *Science* 283 (1999): 1461–1463. These perceptions account for some scientists' estimates that only 5 to 10 percent of their peers are truly interested in communicating with the public. National Cancer Institute, "Scientists' Views on Communicating Cancer Research: Findings from Focus Groups with Intramural Scientists" (Office of Cancer Communications Health Promotions Branch, Bethesda, Maryland, 1998, photocopy), p. iii.

79. Barbara Jasny, R. Brooks Hanson, and Floyd Bloom, "A Media Uncertainty Principle," *Science* 283 (1999): 1453.

80. Shuchman and Wilkes, "Medical Scientists," p. 981

81. Matthew Kieran, *Media Ethics: A Philosophical Approach* (Westport, Connecticut: Praeger, 1997).

82. National Academy of Sciences, *On Being a Scientist: Responsible Conduct in Research*, 2d ed. (Washington, DC: National Academy Press, 1995).

83. Sarah Edwards, et al., "Informed Consent for Clinical Trials: In Search of the 'Best' Method," *Social Science and Medicine* 47 (1998): 1825–1840. These authors conclude that the "more that patients know *before* they are invited to participate in a trial, the better equipped they are to cope with the informed consent procedure." Ibid., p. 1825.

84. Nelkin, *Selling Science*, pp. 161–163.

85. Jane Weeks, et al., "Relationship Between Cancer Patients' Predictions of Prognosis and Their Treatment Preferences," *Journal of the American Medical Association* 279 (1998): 1709–1714.

86. A case in Italy is a prime example. In 1997, numerous media stories reported favorably on a physician's unproven approach to treating cancer that failed to respond to conventional therapies. The stories fueled high patient demand and a campaign to secure state coverage for the costs of the regimen, which was eventually shown to be

ineffective. Rodolfo Pasalacqua, et al., "Patients' Opinions, Feelings, and Attitudes After a Campaign to Promote the Di Bella Therapy," *Lancet* 353 (1999): 1310–1314.

87. Roberto Grilli, "Media Have Key Role in Shaping Use of Health Services," *British Medical Journal* 319 (1999): 786–787.

88. Rebecca Crandall, "Research Funding and the Media," *Journal of the American Medical Association* 266 (1991): 1279, 1282.

89. See chapter 1 for a discussion of the therapeutic misconception.

90. Jasny, Hanson, and Bloom, "Media Uncertainty," p. 1453.

91. National Health Council, *21st Century Housecall*, p. 9.

92. Spyros Andreopoulos, "Hype Hurts Science," *New York Times*, 7 May 1998, A34.

93. Jon Turney, "Public Understanding of Science," *Lancet* 347 (1996): 1087–1090.

94. Ibid., p. 1090. This attitude is exemplified in a scientist's congressional testimony about the need to improve popular reporting on science: "As I gained more experience talking with the public [about animal research], I realized that the public was eager to learn the facts, and once they had the facts, they usually came out on the appropriate side of the issue." House of Representatives Committee on Science, *Communicating Science and Engineering in a Sound-Bite World*, 14 May 1998. Statement of Stuart Zola accessible on the Internet at http://www.house.gov/science/zola_05–14htm.

95. "Communicating Science to the Public: Whose Job Is It Anyway?" *Journal of the National Cancer Institute* 90 (1998): 1509–1511.

96. Wilkie, "Sources in Science," pp. 1309–1310.

97. Shapiro, "Pushing the 'Cure,' " p. 15.

98. Ibid., p. 16.

99. Harvey Fineberg and Sylvia Rowe, "Improving Public Understanding: Guidelines for Communicating Emerging Science on Nutrition, Food Safety, and Health," *Journal of the National Cancer Institute* 90 (1998): 194–199.

100. Ibid., p. 197.

101. Shuchman and Wilkes, "Medical Scientists," pp. 978–979.

102. Angell and Kassirer, "Clinical Research," p. 190.

103. Fineberg and Rowe, "Improving Public Understanding," p. 195.

104. Winsten, "Science and the Media," p. 21.

105. Angell and Kassirer, "Clinical Research," p. 190.

106. Fineberg and Rowe, "Improving Public Understanding," p. 195.

107. Ibid., p. 196.

108. Ibid., p. 197.

109. Joel Greenberg, "Using Sources," in ed. Blum and Knudson, *Field Guide*, pp. 94–101.

110. Fineberg and Rowe, "Improving Public Understanding," p. 196.

111. Lawrence Altman, "Good News From the Front in the War Against Cancer," *New York Times*, 26 May 1998, B10.

112. Shuchman and Wilkes, "Medical Scientists," p. 978.

113. Hartz and Chappell, *Worlds Apart*, p. 93.

114. Ibid.

115. Boyce Rensberger, "Covering Science for Newspapers," in ed. Blum and Knudson, *Field Guide*, pp. 7–16.

116. Eliot Marshall, "The Power of the Front Page of the *New York Times*," *Science* 280 (1998): 996–997.

117. James Watson, "High Hopes on Cancer," *New York Times,* 7 May 1998, A34.

118. Richard Deyo, et al., "The Messenger Under Attack—Intimidation of Re-

searchers By Special-Interest Groups," *New England Journal of Medicine* 336 (1997): 1176–1180.

119. Hartz and Chappell, *Worlds Apart*, p. 108.

120. Ibid., pp. 96–97.

121. Turney, "Public Understanding," p. 1088.

122. Winsten, "Science and the Media," p. 22.

123. Entwhistle, "Reporting Research," p. 922.

124. Deyo et al., "Messenger Under Attack," p. 1178.

125. Angell and Kassirer, "Clinical Research," p. 189.

126. Jerry Canary, "Fighting Cancer," *Indianapolis Star,* 19 May 1998, A9.

127. Barry Bloom, "News About Cancer: What's Fit to Print," *Hastings Center Report* 9 (August 1979): 7.

128. David Resnik, *The Ethics of Science: An Introduction* (New York: Routledge, 1998), pp. 119–21.

129. Shuchman and Wilkes, "Medical Scientists," p. 977.

130. Mary Ellen Sheridan, "The University Community and the A-110 Proposed Revision," 1999. American Association for the Advancement of Science-Federal Focus: Briefing on Data Access, accessible on the Internet at http://www.aaas.org/spp/dspp/sfrl/projects/omb/sheridan.htm.

131. Paul Friedman, "Mistakes and Fraud in Medical Research," *Law, Medicine & Health Care* 20 (1992): 17–25.

132. Johnson, "Shattuck Lecture," p. 90.

133. Tony Delamothe and Richard Smith, "Moving Beyond Journals: The Future Arrives With a Crash," *British Medical Journal* 318 (1999): 1637–1639.

134. In 1998, these issues were widely debated in the context of a proposal to create a government Website that would permit studies to be posted after a quick check by one or two experts. Opponents argued that including clinical research in this system could have a substantial negative impact on the public. Arnold Relman, "The NIH 'E-Biomed' Proposal—A Potential Threat to the Evaluation and Orderly Dissemination of New Clinical Studies," *New England Journal of Medicine* 340 (1999): 1828–29. One electronic archive tries to avoid misleading the public by attaching prominent warnings to every study that has not been accepted by a peer-reviewed journal. Tony Delamothe, et al., "Netprints: The Next Phase in the Evolution of Biomedical Publishing," *British Medical Journal* 319 (1999): 1515–1516.

135. Margaret Winkler and Phil Fontanarosa, "JAMA-EXPRESS: Rapid Peer Review and Publication," *Journal of the American Medical Association* 281 (1999): 1754–1755.

136. Delamothe and Smith, "Moving Beyond Journals," p. 1638.

137. See, for example, Robert Golden, "Serotonin and Depression," *National Depressive and Manic Depressive Association Outreach Newsletter,* Winter 1999: 6.

138. See, for example, National Breast Cancer Coalition. Accessible on the Internet at http://www.natlbcc.org.

139. See Robert Finn, *Cancer Clinical Trials: Experimental Treatments and How They Can Help You* (Sebastopol, California: O'Reilly, 1999), pp. 164–166.

140. Donald Earl Henson, "Cancer and the Internet," *Cancer* 86 (1999): 373–374.

141. Sasha Shepperd, Deborah Charnock, and Bob Gann, "Helping Patients Access High-Quality Health Information," *British Medical Journal* 319 (1999): 764–766.

142. National Health Council, "Key Survey Findings," 1997. Accessible on the Internet at http://healthanswers.com/sources/nhc/21st_century/21st_housecall-2.asp.

143. In describing the advocacy efforts of Christopher Reeve, for example, columnist Tony Snow wrote that Reeve "describes progress as if he were talking about ordering a burger carry-out: All we need to do, he says, is 'pay for a cure.' " Tony Snow, "Reeve Talks to the Wrong Guys," *Cleveland Plain Dealer*, 22 March 1998, 1-D.

144. Giuseppe Remuzzi and Arrigo Schieppati, "Lessons From the Di Bella Affair," *Lancet* 353 (1999): 1290–1291. In a well-known U.S. example, the film *Lorenzo's Oil* mixed parent–advocates' enthusiasm with Hollywood drama to suggest that an untested substance effectively treated a child's life-threatening genetic disorder. Research later found that the substance conferred no benefit. Ronald Wanders, "A Happier Sequel to *Lorenzo's Oil*?" *Nature Medicine* 4 (1998): 1245–1246. After the film, some parents who tried the oil reportedly were "bitterly disappointed with the treatment and angry that the movie depicted it as a cure." Gina Kolata, "Lorenzo's Oil: A Movie Outruns Science," *New York Times*, 9 February 1993, C1, C6.

145. Fineberg and Rowe, "Improving Public Understanding," p. 197.

146. Efforts to institute a system of quality control are described in Charles Marwick, "Ensuring Ethical Internet Information," *Journal of the American Medical Association* 283 (2000): 1677–1678 and Margaret A. Winkler, et al., "Guidelines for Medical and Health Information Sites on the Internet," *Journal of the American Medical Association* 283 (2000): 1600–1606.

147. Mi Young Hwang, "Navigating the Maze of Medical Research," *Journal of the American Medical Association* 280 (1998): 306.

148. Aniruddha Malpani, "Health Library in India Works to Empower Patients," *British Medical Journal* 319 (1999): 785.

149. Rebecca Dresser, "Surfing for Studies," *Hastings Center Report* 29 (November-December 1999): pp. 26–27.

150. Alzheimer's Association, "Caution Urged Regarding Newly Published Research on Caloric Intake and Brain Disorders," 4 January 1999. Accessible on the Internet, at http://www.alz.org/news/rtcaloric.htm.

151. National Health Council, *21st Century Housecall*, p. 12.

152. National Breast Cancer Coalition, "Workshops for the Media: Understanding Breast Cancer Science and Policy," 1999. Accessible on the Internet at http://www.natlbcc.org/meetings/mediaw/wftm_sciencepolicy.asp.

153. Angell and Kassirer, "Clinical Research," pp. 189–190.

154. John Adams, "Argument in Defense of the Soldiers in the Boston Massacre Trials," in *Bartlett's Familiar Quotations*, ed. Justin Kaplan, 16th ed. (Boston: Little, Brown and Company, 1992).

Chapter 8

1. Mary Woolley, "Advocacy for Health Research Means Advocacy for Patient Care," *Nursing Outlook* 45 (1997): 44.

2. Vida Foubister, "Research Reservations," *American Medical News*, 31 (January 2000): 8–10.

3. Barbara Katz Rothman, *Genetic Maps and Human Imaginations* (New York: W. W. Norton & Company, 1998), p. 38.

4. Katherine Russell Rich, "Close to the Bone," *New York Times Magazine*, 19 December 1999, 102.

5. A review of research contributions to treating and preventing heart disease is provided in Stephen Klaidman, *Saving the Heart* (New York: Oxford University Press, 2000), pp. 221–222.

6. Daniel Callahan, "Death and the Research Imperative," *New England Journal of Medicine* 342 (2000): 654–656.

7. Ibid., p. 655.

8. Bernard Lo, *Resolving Ethical Dilemmas: A Guide for Clinicians* (Baltimore, Maryland: Williams & Wilkins, 1995), pp. 56–63.

9. Jane Poulson, "Bitter Pills to Swallow," *New England Journal of Medicine* 338 (1998): 1844–1846.

10. Nicholas A. Christakis, *Death Foretold: Prophecy and Prognosis in Medical Care* (Chicago: University of Chicago Press, 1999).

11. These programs are discussed in chapter 3.

12. Alisa Harrison, "All Change?" *British Medical Journal* 319 (1999): 793.

13. I thank Carl Wellman for alerting me to these issues.

14. Bruce C. Wolpe and Bertram J. Levine, *Lobbying Congress: How the System Works* (Washington, DC: Congressional Quarterly, 1996), pp. 27–28.

15. Ibid., p. 26.

16. *Codes of Professional Responsibility*, ed. Rena A. Gorlin, 3d ed. (Washington, DC: Bureau of National Affairs, 1994).

17. Amy Gutmann and Dennis Thompson, *Democracy and Disagreement* (Cambridge, Massachusetts: Harvard University Press, 1996), pp. 144–151.

18. David Luban, *Lawyers and Justice: An Ethical Study* (Princeton, New Jersey: Princeton University Press, 1988), pp. 11–30.

19. Luban, *Lawyers and Justice*, p. 378 (citing Heidi Garland, "Lawyers as Lobbyists: Auto Safety Regulation," Harvard Law School Program on the Legal Profession Case Study PLP-83–012, 27 October 1983, p. 19).

20. Gutmann and Thompson, *Democracy and Disagreement*, pp. 128–164.

21. Luban, *Lawyers and Justice*, pp. 50–174.

22. Steven Epstein, *Impure Science: AIDS, Activism, and the Politics of Knowledge* (Berkeley: University of California Press, 1996), pp.105–178.

23. Ibid., pp. 287–294, 352–353.

24. Benjamin Freedman, "The Ethics and Politics of Human Experimentation" (Book Review), *New England Journal of Medicine* 329 (1993):1748.

25. Alison Miller, "Trial Run," *American Medical News*, 27 September 1999, 17–18.

26. Kurt Eichenwald and Gina Kolata, "Drug Trials Hide Conflicts for Doctors," *New York Times*, 16 May 1999, A1, A28–A29.

27. Vida Foubister, "Clinical Trial Pay Troubling Topic at CEJA Forum," American Medical News, 27 December 1999, 8–9.

28. Eichenwald and Kolata, "Drug Trials," A28.

29. Ibid., p. A28.

30. Stuart E. Lind, "Finder's Fees for Research Subjects," *New England Journal of Medicine* 323 (1990): 192–195.

31. Department of Health and Human Services Office of Inspector General, *Institutional Review Boards: A Time for Reform*, OEI-01–97-00193 (Washington, DC: Government Printing Office, 1998), pp. 5–6.

32. Troyen A. Brennan, "Proposed Revisions to the Declaration of Helsinki—Will They Weaken the Ethical Principles Underlying Human Research?" *New England Journal of Medicine* 341 (1999): 527–531.

33. Department of Health and Human Services Office of Inspector General, *Institutional Review Boards: The Emergence of Independent Boards*, OEI-01–97-00192 (Washington, DC: Government Printing Office, 1998).

34. Thomas Bodenheimer, "Uneasy Alliance: Clinical Investigators and the Pharmaceutical Industry," *New England Journal of Medicine* 342 (2000): 1539–1544.

35. Mildred Cho and Lisa Bero, "The Quality of Drug Studies Published in Symposium Proceedings," *Annals of Internal Medicine* 124 (1996): 485–489.

36. Drummond Rennie, "Thyroid Storm," *Journal of the American Medical Association* 277 (1997): 1238–1243.

37. David Blumenthal, et al., "Withholding Research Results in Academic Life Sciences," *Journal of the American Medical Association* 277 (1997): 1224–1228.

38. Ezekiel Emanuel and Daniel Steiner, "Institutional Conflict of Interest," *New England Journal of Medicine* 332 (1995): 262–267.

39. Eichenwald and Kolata, "Drug Trials," p. A29.

40. Paul T. Kefalides, "Research on Humans Faces Scrutiny; New Policies Adopted," *Annals of Internal Medicine* 132 (2000): 513–516.

41. Rebecca Dresser, "Time for New Rules on Human Subjects Research?" *Hastings Center Report* 28 (November-December 1998): 23–24.

42. Economist Julianne Malveaux argues that breast cancer advocates have the economic clout to make corporations more responsive to patients' needs. Mary Ann Swissler, "An Economist Looks at the Price of Awareness," *Breast Cancer Action*, January-February 2000, p. 3.

43. Marcia Angell, "The Pharmaceutical Industry—To Whom Is It Accountable?" *New England Journal of Medicine* 342 (2000): 1902–1904.

44. See Martin Enserink, "Radical Steps Urged to Help Underserved," *Science* 288 (2000): 1563–1564 and Martin Enserink, "Group Urges Action on Third World Drugs," *Science* 287 (2000): 1571.

45. Jon Cohen, "Philanthropy's Rising Tide Lifts Science," *Science* 286 (1999): 214–223.

46. Meyer Rangell, "The Uses of Wealth, Public and Private," *New York Times*, 17 September 1999, A26.

47. Reed Abelson, "Sales Pitches Tied to Charities Draw States' Scrutiny," *New York Times*, 3 May 1999, A1, A20.

48. Institute of Medicine, *Xenotransplantation: Science, Ethics, and Public Policy* (Washington, DC: National Academy Press, 1996), pp. 57–61.

49. Daniel Perry, "Patients' Voices: The Powerful Sound in the Stem Cell Debate," *Science* 287 (2000): 1423.

50. Vida Foubister, "Intense Scrutiny Confronts Gene Therapy," *American Medical News*, 28 February 2000, pp. 1, 26.

51. Jeremy Sugarman, "Ethical Considerations in Leaping from Bench to Bedside," *Science* 285 (1999): 2071–2072.

52. Institute of Medicine, *Xenotransplantation*, pp. 39–56.

53. John Harris, "Intimations of Immortality," *Science* 288 (2000): 59.

54. Council on Ethical and Judicial Affairs, American Medical Association, "Ethical Issues Related to Prenatal Genetic Screening," *Archives of Family Medicine* 3 (1994): 633–642.

55. Jon W. Gordon, "Genetic Enhancement in Humans," *Science* 283 (1999): 2023–2024.

56. Claudia Dreifus, "Still Living With AIDS, and Endless Jokes About Bananas," *New York Times*, 13 October 1998, D3.

57. Vida Foubister, "Gene Therapy Fosters Hope," *American Medical News*, 6 March 2000, pp. 10, 12–13.

58. Perry, "Patients' Voices," p. 1423.

59. Theodore Friedman, "Principles for Human Gene Studies," *Science* 287 (2000): 2163–2165.

60. Nicholas Wade, "Cancer Society Quits Group on Cell Research," *New York Times*, 29 July 1999, A18.

61. Ezekiel Emanuel, "A Phase I Trial on the Ethics of Phase I Trials," *Journal of Clinical Oncology* 13 (1995): 1049–1051.

62. Maureen Dowd, "W., in the Pink," *New York Times*, 5 March 2000, A19.

63. Richard Deyo et al., "The Messenger Under Attack—Intimidation of Researchers By Special-Interest Groups," *New England Journal of Medicine* 336 (1997): 1176–1180.

INDEX

Academic freedom of researchers, 34–35, 41–42

Access
  to experimental interventions, 46–70, 108, 153–54, 156, 159–63, 166, 200–01 n.86
  to health care, 9, 47, 64–65, 69–70, 154, 162–63, 171–72

Accountability principle in deliberative democracy, 100

Activists. *See* Breast cancer advocates; HIV/ AIDS advocates; Patient advocates

Adolescent health research, 81

Advertisements
  for medical products, 137–38, 140, 149
  for research, 119, 197 n.75
  for research participants, 58, 67

Advisory Committee on Human Radiation Experiments, 56–57, 59

Advocates. *See* Community; Patient advocates; Representation

"Affirmative action" in research funding, 82, 84

African Americans in research, 13, 102

Aggregation problem in allocating resources, 82

AIDS activists. *See* HIV/AIDS advocates

"AIDS backlash," 98

AIDS research. *See* HIV/AIDS, research on

Alcoholism, research on 115

Alexander, Leo, 14–15

Altruism and research, 30, 57, 67, 108

Alzheimer's disease research, 49, 63, 145.
  See also Dementia, research on

American Cancer Society, 133

American College of Radiology, 133

American Heart Association, 94

American League of Lobbyists, 105–06, 163

American Medical Association, 85

Angiostatin, 132, 136, 143, 145, 198 n.16

Animal studies, 114–15, 131–32, 144, 146, 170

Arthritis, research on, 82

Ashkenazi Jewish groups, 115

Australia, research review system, 115, 121–22

Authorship in participatory research, 35

Autonomy in research decision making, 52, 55–60, 67–68, 140, 146, 158. *See also* Informed decisions

Bazell, Robert, 186 n.100

Belmont Report, 12–14, 157

Beneficence principle in research, 13, 29–31
  and ethics review, 117
  and expanded access to experimental interventions, 53–54, 60–63, 68–69

Benefits of research. *See* Beneficence principle in research; Research, goals of

Bioethics
  field of, ix-xi, 18
  in research ethics review, 120, 125
  relationship to advocacy, ix, 12, 15, 156–59

Biomedical research. *See* Research

Birth defects, research on, 75

"Bottom-up" approach to ethics and standards, 144, 158

Breakthroughs in research, 6, 17, 67–68, 70, 132, 135, 138, 143–44, 150

Breast cancer activists. *See* Breast cancer advocates

Breast cancer advocates, 6, 15, 104, 156, 174 n.21
  and access to experimental interventions, 58, 62, 66
  and research funding, 36, 74, 94, 96–97
  in research merit review, 25–26

207

Phase I cancer trials, 56–58, 68, 171

Physicians' discussions of research, 50, 57–58, 132, 139–41, 146

Placebos in research, 24–25, 30–31, 56–58, 61, 183–84 n.48

Pneumonia, research on, 84

"Political correctness" and research, 6, 33, 62, 79, 155

Politics and research funding, 5, 17, 75–76, 87, 99, 160, 171

Poor-quality research, 97–98, 147, 155, 168

Popular media, 74
    as sources of research information, 5, 17, 58, 67–68, 130–50, 156, 160–61, 197 n.4, 200–01 n.86, 201 n.94

Porter, John, 94

Poverty, research on diseases of, 81, 98, 156

Prediction of research applications, 78–79, 82–83

President's budget for National Institutes of Health, 75–76

Press releases and conferences about research, 133, 137, 142, 144

Prevention, research on, 75, 80–81, 134

Priority setting for federally funded research, 73–90
    criteria for, 75–77, 87
    criticism of, 79–80
    process for, 77–78
    proposed revisions in, 79–80, 87–90
    public participation in, 78–80, 89–90, 92–108. See also National Institutes of Health (NIH)

Private foundations and research funding. See Foundation funding for research

Procedural justice
    public perceptions of, 85–86, 100
    in research decisions, 156
    in research funding system, 87–90, 100–103, 107
    in resource allocation, 16, 80, 85–89

Professional interest groups, 106, 133–34

Professional myopia in research review, 116, 154

Prostate cancer, research on, 47, 76, 94, 97

Psychiatric research. See Mental illness, research on

Public health needs, evaluation of, 7, 16, 76–77, 79, 108

Public image of science, 77, 87, 89, 136, 139–42, 154

Public participation
    in research ethics oversight, 17, 111–28
    in research priority setting, 75, 89–90, 93–108. See also Community; Consumers; Patient advocates

Public relations
    and patient advocacy, 171
    and public participation, 36, 103, 116–20
    and research reporting, 130

Public release of research findings, 138, 145–48

Public trust in research system, 117–19, 139, 141

Public understanding of research, 126, 141–42, 144–45, 149–50

Publication of research findings, 34–35, 42, 137–38, 147

Publicity principle in deliberative democracy, 100

Randomization in research, 23, 56, 117, 183–84 n.48

Randomized clinical trial, 14, 23–25, 62

Rare diseases, research on, 82, 169

Realistic perspective on research advances, need for, xi, 8, 159–61, 166, 171–72
    in advocacy for expanded access, 48, 59, 66, 70
    in ethics review, 126–28
    in reporting on research, 18, 131, 140, 146
    in research priority setting, 80

Reciprocity principle, in deliberative democracy, 100

Reeve, Christopher, 203 n.143

Regulatory system for research, 14, 50, 55–56, 111–28

Rehnquist, William H., 85

Religion and research, 17, 27, 85, 116, 119

Reporting on research findings, 130–50
    advocates and, 17–18, 131, 133, 141–50
    journalists and, 132–36, 139–41, 153–56
    problems with, 17, 58, 70, 130–41
    proposed reforms, 141–45, 148–50

Representation
    of constituents, 10, 36, 40, 156, 169, 180 n.100
    of public, 7, 86, 103, 105–06, 112–15, 117–18, 128, 157–58, 164
    of research participants, 42, 113–15, 117–18, 122–23, 127, 180 n.110, 194 n.9, 197 n.80
    problems in, 36–39, 42, 105–06, 118, 122–23, 127, 161–62, 166–67

Representative government, 101, 105

Representatives. See Community; Patient advocates; Representation

Reproductive risks in research, 50, 53

Research
    advances, nature of, 6, 9, 63, 66, 70, 81–